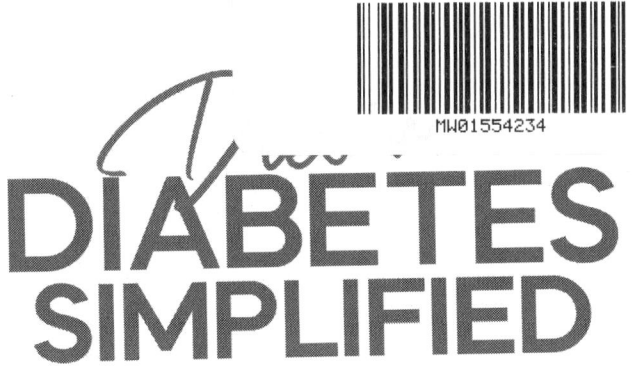

DIABETES SIMPLIFIED

Your Personal Diabetes Nutrition Coach

SHERYL SALIS

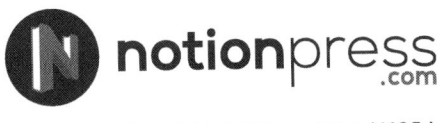

INDIA · SINGAPORE · MALAYSIA

Notion Press

Old No. 38, New No. 6
McNichols Road, Chetpet
Chennai - 600 031

First Published by Notion Press 2020
Copyright © Sheryl Salis 2020
All Rights Reserved.

ISBN 978-1-64587-868-1

This book has been published with all efforts taken to make the material error-free after the consent of the author. However, the author and the publisher do not assume and hereby disclaim any liability to any party for any loss, damage, or disruption caused by errors or omissions, whether such errors or omissions result from negligence, accident, or any other cause.

While every effort has been made to avoid any mistake or omission, this publication is being sold on the condition and understanding that neither the author nor the publishers or printers would be liable in any manner to any person by reason of any mistake or omission in this publication or for any action taken or omitted to be taken or advice rendered or accepted on the basis of this work. For any defect in printing or binding the publishers will be liable only to replace the defective copy by another copy of this work then available.

Contents

Foreword 5

Acknowledgements 11

1. Nutrition Basics 13
2. Are You in the Safe Zone? – Let's Find Out 31
3. Proteins 37
4. Fats and Oils 43
5. The Carb Story 61
6. The Story of Numbers: Glycemic Index and Glycemic Load 79
7. Hypothyroidism and Its Dietary Management 95
8. Hyperuricemia (High Uric Acid Levels) 97
9. All about Carbohydrate, Protein and Fat Counting 101
10. Hypoglycaemia 121
11. Gestational Diabetes Mellitus (GDM) 133

12.	Exercise	151
13.	Get Label Wise	159
14.	Eating out Options	179
15.	Smart Cooking	195
16.	Superfoods	205
17.	Healthy Recipes	215

Testimonials 229

Foreword

It gives me great pleasure to write a foreword for such an educative and enlightening book on one of the main pillars of diabetes management – Nutrition. Somehow, nutrition, which is a vital aspect of maintenance of health, is the most neglected one. Along with education, nutrition forms the basis to self-manage one's diabetes.

Unfortunately the medical profession is prevented from learning the science of nutrition as it is included in the subject of preventive medicine. Hence medical caregivers are unable to provide proper nutritional guidance to the patients and their family. This is where this book will help fill the gap and make the patient and one's family self-reliant in one aspect of diabetes management.

There is a real need of a good book on nutrition. In today's world, our nutrition is dominated by commercial sources with the help of advertisements on TV and newspapers. Home cooked food and traditional cooking has been replaced by the food available online. This has led to different metabolic disorders being present in increased numbers in the population. Such disorders have started surpassing the number of persons suffering from infectious diseases. And this is all due to faulty lifestyle.

Nutrition plays an important role in faulty lifestyle. The onslaught of western commercial foods and soft drinks and their modified counterparts of vadapav, etc. as our major nutritional intake along with a sedentary and stressful lifestyle have added to the problems. Unfortunately in our society there are many so called nutrition experts without proper qualifications who bombard the gullible society with their nutritional fads without any scientific background.

In the field of diabetology, nutrition is the first and the most important step in its management. Sheryl Salis, with her years of both theoretical and practical experience in the field of nutrition has written a very practical and easily understandable book on nutrition. She has poured out her experience of dealing with all types of individuals with diabetes but especially so for those having type 1 diabetes who either are on a multi dose intensive insulin therapy or on an insulin pump. She has made carbohydrate counting and other nutritional aspects for basal bolus insulin regimes an easy process. Thereby the patients can completely control their diabetes even at a very young age and lead an exceptionally active and fruitful life. I am sure this book will be welcomed by all the individuals with diabetes in India to make their day to day living happy and healthy.

Having covered most of the practical problems in day to day life one should be a self-reliant person with the help of this book. This book would also be a great help to the busy medical practitioners to guide people with diabetes. Sheryl has done her job as a dedicated, experienced and at the same time understanding humane nutritional counsellor and provided a gold mine for them to gather the nuggets of nutritional wisdom. The map has been laid down it is up to you to chart your course.

– By Dr. Vijay S. Ajgaonkar
Consultant Diabetologist, Mumbai
Founder: Juvenile Diabetes Foundation, Maharashtra Chapter.

A *simplified* book on *diet in diabetes* by an *Indian* author has been a long felt need. The title of this book is very apt as diet is always considered a complex issue by patients as well as the treating physicians.

As a paediatric diabetologist, I deal with diabetes only in the below 18 years age group. In this group, over 95% have type 1 diabetes while type 2 diabetes is very rare. Most books on diet in diabetes discuss type 2 diabetes at length but do not highlight the major differences in dietary needs of children and adolescents with type 1 diabetes.

Those in the pediatric group do not need a "diet" in the restrictive sense. They are in the growing phase and hence must eat as much as any non-diabetic youth of the same age and sex. However, they need to eat "healthy". They must be taught what foods are "healthy" and what is "unhealthy" or "junk food". Their family members too should be convinced to eat only the right foods. They must be made to understand that eating is for providing good fuel to the body and not for pleasure or entertainment. Unhealthy foods unfortunately taste better and can provide one's calorie needs but in the long term they harm the human body.

An important aim of diabetes management in childhood and adolescence is to ensure that they enjoy a normal life and hence, they should not be expected to modify their lifestyle to accommodate a diet prescription. A fixed diet prescription has *no role* in children and adolescents with diabetes. Instead, they should be allowed to eat whenever their school and play timings permit so that they do not feel different from their peers. To ensure that this does not disrupt their blood sugars they have to be taught how to modify their pre-meal insulin bolus dose to match the timing and carbohydrate content of meals. The concept of carbohydrate counting is very important and this must be taught from the outset.

Children cannot be stopped from participating in unplanned physical activities. They should receive guidance on selecting appropriate snacks before such activities to prevent hypoglycaemia.

When children are unwell they lose their appetite and eat very little but at the same time they have high levels of stress hormones in the body so that blood sugars (and ketones) tend to go haywire: either very high or very low. They can also get acidotic and dehydrated. Written instructions must be provided on what they can eat or drink when they are unwell and anorexic so that their sugars and hydration are maintained.

Finally, children cannot be expected to be perfect saints. They will at times succumb to temptation and peer pressure and consume "junk" foods. How they can "sin" *once in a while* and yet maintain blood glucose, is another aspect that must be taught but not encouraged.

I am pleased to note that all these aspects are brought out brilliantly in this book. I have known Sheryl Salis for many years. Her knowledge, her quest for improvement and innovation, her flair for teaching and her genuine interest in helping patients with juvenile diabetes are admirable. This book is a must read for all patients as well as doctors and nutritionists.

– Dr. Aspi J. Irani. MD, DCH.
Consultant: Nanavati Super Speciality Hospital, Mumbai.
Trustee: Juvenile Diabetes Foundation, Maharashtra Chapter.

"Annam Parabrahmaha Swaroopam" and "Annam Aushadham" are phrases in Sanskrit Vedic literature which highlight the importance of food, meaning "Food is a reflection of god" and "Food is medicine", as opposed to food that is eaten only to satisfy the tastebuds. A lot of illnesses are linked to correct or incorrect food intake, and therefore, a working knowledge of diet is very essential for every human being.

As true as this is, in no other field do I find it more important than in the world of diabetes, in my experience as a Paediatric Endocrinologist with 12 years of European expertise and many in India.

In diabetes, whether type 1 or type 2, whether in adults or in children, diet is a very important part of treatment just as medicines are. The ability to know what is in your diet and how it will affect your blood sugars and therefore how to adjust medications is very important. Also equally important is what to eat and in what quantities.

The families I meet are usually stunned with the diagnosis, and from thereon, undergo a crash course in diet specifics. In addition, is the fact that Indian diets are very varied. For example, a sambar (a kind of lentil curry) can vary widely based on how it is prepared. This tends to make things more tricky for families.

However, this book by Ms. Sheryl Salis, is very much welcome. Ms. Salis, with her superior expertise, and her practical and patient-friendly manner, makes the job of diet in diabetes truly what the title suggests, 'Simplified'.

From my experience, everyone with diabetes should really take out the time to go and consult Ms. Salis and use the book as an adjunct/aid to back up what is discussed in the consultation. This is because a good understanding of diet in diabetes is a real foundation for the future, not just for the patient, but also for the rest of the family to move toward healthy eating habits.

If meeting Ms. Salis is not possible, even the book in itself is one of the best there is out in the market.

– Dr. Smita Koppikar
Consultant Paediatric Endocrinologist
Mumbai, India

Acknowledgements

This book is a labour of love and a tribute to my late father Mr. George Salis who left us for his heavenly abode twenty five years ago. He has been my role model and inspiration in serving and contributing to the society at large.

This book would not have been possible without the support of my family especially my mother Mrs. Cecilia Salis, husband Dr. Peter Fernandez and son Ethan Fernandez who have been very patient and understanding given the time I spent researching and writing this book.

I would like to thank my parent, mentor and guide Dr. V S Ajgaonkar for his persuasion, constant encouragement and motivation to write this book. The idea of writing this book came from him.

Heartfelt gratitude to Dr. Aspi J Irani and Dr. Smita Koppikar for their patient reading, timely feedback and valuable inputs.

My deepest gratitude to the entire team who have helped make this book possible.

First and foremost Mrs. Seema Verma, (founder of Content Junction) who readily agreed to edit this book and whose invaluable contributions and inputs have made this book an interesting read.

Senior dieticians Ms. Shweta Gosalia and Ms. Natasha Vora, for contributing very relevant and interesting chapters on Healthy Recipes and Smart Cooking in this book.

Ms. Preethi Rahul, Ms. Shefa Syed, Ms. Minal Gada & Ms. Sangeeta Costa Correia, for their help in researching, editing and proofreading this book at different stages.

Dr. Prabodh Halde, Ms. Geeta Malhotra, Ms. Bina Chheda, Ms. Subhaprada Nishtala and Ms. Priyal Warty Mayekar for their timely suggestions and relentless support.

Sincere gratitude to all the people (teachers, friends, fraternity and well-wishers) who have been a huge support through the years and have inspired me to do better work.

Last but not least, a big thank you to my dearest patients who have been my biggest teachers and whose experiences have helped shaped this book.

Happy Reading!

– **Sheryl Salis**

CHAPTER 01 Nutrition Basics

When you are diagnosed with diabetes or pre-diabetes, the first thing that comes to mind is that you have to give up your favourite foods. Most people feel that they have lost the sweetness of life because they can no longer indulge in the foods they like.

Food is such an important part of life that when a person is diagnosed with diabetes or pre-diabetes, the mind is more concerned about not being able to enjoy good food rather than being bothered about managing the condition.

Most of the time, young or adult patients shy away from visiting the dietitian because of wrong beliefs. They feel that visiting the dietitian is only about getting restrictions on their food. *Do you also feel the same?*

If so, you need to rethink. With changing times and advancement in the field of research, nutrition experts have also figured out ways to manage the emotions and sensitivities connected to food.

I, as a Dietitian, am often posed with this question, "What should I eat?", "Can I eat fruits?", "What about mangoes, will I never be able to enjoy them?", "I am a rice eater, now that I am diagnosed with diabetes, what should I do?" and many more such questions.

I tell them, "Eat everything." which brings a smile on their face, **BUT** "Watch your portions." ***Rather than focusing on the foods, you need to restrict, think about all the delicious choices you have!*** The variety of foods that you can eat is vast. You need to look at that too.

Food does influence your blood glucose levels. But understanding the right combination and timing of eating various foods can help you manage your blood glucose levels better.

This book will address all your doubts in subsequent chapters.

> It is not only about what you eat, but how much you eat, that matters. Moderation is the key to good health.

Understanding the Food Plate

Understanding the food plate or the food that we eat on a day-to-day basis is important. Food provides important nutrients like carbohydrate, protein, fat, fibre, vitamins and minerals. Choosing from the variety of options from each food group helps ensure that you get the right amounts of all the good nutrients required to maintain good health. This is called Diet Diversity.

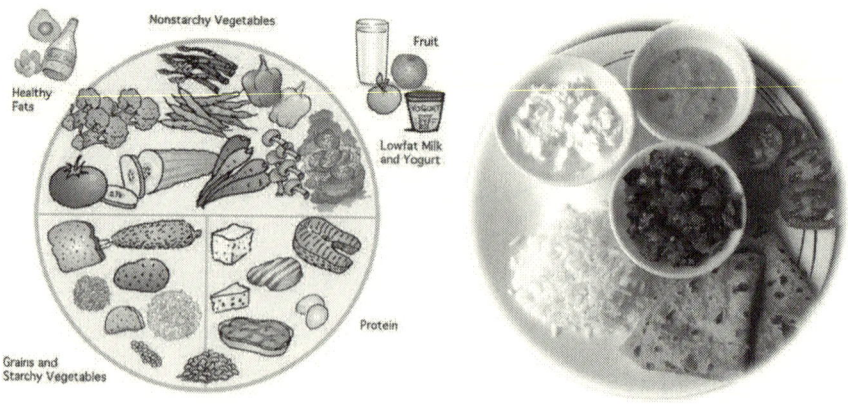

Healthy Food Plate

The Healthy Food Plate

Choose a 9" plate instead of a 12" plate. Fill half the plate with vegetables and salads. Fill 1/4th of the plate with starch and cereals (whole grains, whole wheat flour, broken wheat (daliya), rice, potatoes and root vegetables, millets like ragi/nachni, jowar, bajra) and the remaining 1/4th plate with protein (lean meat, egg, milk, paneer, curd/yogurt, soybean, tofu, dals, whole pulses and sprouts).

Let's Understand the Major Food Groups and Their Role in Maintaining Good Health

Grains and Legumes

This group includes cereals like wheat, rice, jowar, bajra, ragi, quinoa, barley, broken wheat (daliya/lapsi), breakfast cereals, bread, biscuits, oats, noodles, pasta and maida. Pulses such as green gram (moong), kidney beans (rajma), Bengal gram (chana), soybean, cow pea (lobia), chickpeas (white chana), sprouts etc. are also included in this category. Carbohydrates are the most abundant nutrient in this group unlike the common belief that pulses have only protein. Yes, pulses have more protein compared to cereals but they are also sources of carbohydrates. Cereals and pulses alone are not complete protein but when mixed (e.g. Khichdi, dosa, idli: a dal and rice combination) become a complete and good quality protein.

The caloric intake should be higher for a person who does more physical work as compared to a person who has a sedentary lifestyle. Calorie recommendations for each individual would vary based on the weight, activity level, age and other factors.

Meat, Egg, Fish, Milk and Milk products

The Healthy Food Plate encourages you to choose protein sources such as fish, lean meat (de-skinned or skinless chicken), eggs, milk and milk products which provide good quality protein.

Limit the consumption of red meat and avoid processed and canned meat like bacon, sausages, ham and ready to eat products like nuggets, cutlets and kababs as they are high in saturated fat and salt and put you at risk for heart diseases and other metabolic disorders.

For Indians, especially vegetarians, a conscious effort has to be made to add proteins to their daily diet. I have seen that most vegetarians (sometimes non-vegetarians as well) consume very little protein in their diet and are unable to meet their daily protein requirement. A healthy individual is recommended 0.8–1 g protein/kg ideal body weight. It is important to check with a qualified dietitian on your protein requirement for a day.

Milk and milk products from the dairy group are excellent sources of high-quality protein and must be included in every meal. You can include unflavoured or plain yoghurt or curd, buttermilk, whey water (chena paani), and low-fat paneer (cottage cheese) in your daily meal plan. Yogurt is a good source of probiotic and must be included in the diet as it helps to keep the gut healthy. Make sure to consume plain or unflavoured yogurt as flavoured contains added sugar.

Real life example

A 16-year-old boy, Rishabh Shetty (name changed) who was overweight was diagnosed with pre-diabetes (HbA1c-6 %). His neck had a dark black velvety discolouration which indicated that he had insulin resistance. His paediatrician sent him to me for a diet consultation. During consultation, I found that he consumed a high carbohydrate, high-fat diet and there was very little protein intake according to his age and body weight. He would order food from outside often using food delivery apps. His physical activity was minimal and he spent a large part of his free time playing video games. His sleep was inadequate as he was on his phone till late night. The family had a very erratic lifestyle and each of the members in the family were busy doing their own thing.

The family was counselled on the importance of a healthy lifestyle and how parents need to be good role models for their children, I counselled him on the importance of exercise and adequate sleep.

I made changes to his meals by cutting down on the carbs, improved the quality of carbs by restricting refined carb intake and adding whole grains and legumes (dals), added a protein source to every meal so that his body would get adequate protein and the much needed satiety. I also added healthy fats in the form of nuts and seeds for in between snacking. I asked him to refrain from ordering food from out for at least three months. He went home and followed the new meal plan religiously, worked out daily as advised and slept for a good 7 hours every night. He was happy as there were new options added to his meal plan along with his regular food. (*Who said healthy food cannot be yummy?*☺)

His parents were overjoyed as his HbA1c came down to 5.4% in just 3 months and he was now much fitter and energetic than before

It is now a common trend to see kids as young as 10 and 12 years with pre-diabetes and diabetes, thanks to the modern lifestyle – unhealthy eating, no physical activity, lack of sleep and increased screen time, gadget use is pre-disposing our kids to these lifestyle diseases.

Vegetables

The vegetable group comprises of green leafy vegetables, other vegetables and root vegetables. Most vegetables being low in calories and carbohydrates are rich in fibre and micro-nutrients such as vitamin C, folic acid, vitamin B complex, iron and calcium.

Root vegetables such as potato, tapioca, yam and colocasia root are higher in calories and carbohydrates compared to other vegetables. They need to be accounted for in the total carbohydrate budget for the day. Even when you choose a particular vegetable, the way it is cooked has an effect on your blood glucose levels. (Refer to the chapter on glycemic index).

> For instance, a baked jacket potato (potato with skin, cooked and cooled) is preferred over a mashed potato that rapidly increases the blood glucose levels.

Make sure you have vegetables/salads/unstrained vegetable soup with every meal. You can consider having freshly prepared unstrained vegetable juice in the morning to kick start your day, and include unstrained vegetable soup, grilled vegetables, stir fry vegetables in your lunch and dinner to make sure you are meeting your fibre, vitamin and mineral requirements.

Add a dash of colour to your plate by including red, orange and green coloured vegetables in grilled form or as a simple stir fry. This will not only help you meet your fibre, vitamin and mineral requirements but also provide you with the necessary antioxidants (nutrients that fight toxins in the body).

Fruits

Don't fall prey to myths like, "I cannot eat fruits because I have diabetes." Fruits are excellent sources of vitamins, minerals and fibre, which are vital for good health.

Real life example

I met a 45-year-old marketing head of an MNC who needed help in getting his diet planned to manage his erratic work timings and his sugar levels. After a long discussion about his schedule and eating habits, I suggested, "You should eat a fruit in between your meals to avoid long gaps between meals." He was taken aback with the suggestion and said, "I have diabetes, how can I eat fruits? They are sweet and will mess up my blood glucose levels." Expecting this common question, I counselled him. "The good news is that you can eat all sorts of fruits. You can choose from a variety of colourful seasonal fruits. All fruits are not the same. Some fruits are higher in calories than others of the same weight. In such cases, you need to keep a check on the portion of the fruit you eat. For instance, you can choose to eat a small apple or exchange it with a small banana or a medium-sized guava, or kiwi or orange or peach. You can also have 2 small plums, 1 apple, or 1 bowl of melon as a mid-meal snack. Eat a fruit which fits your fist. For example, if you buy apples and get six apples in a kilo, choose smaller ones where you may get eight. This way you get more and eat the right amount.

One word of advice here is to avoid eating fruits immediately after a meal which is usually the practice. Fruits contain fructose, hence, when had with a meal or immediately after a meal increases the carbohydrate load of the meal which in turn leads to an increase in blood glucose levels and triglycerides. It is best to have fruit in the morning as soon as you wake up or as a mid-morning or a mid-evening snack. This will ensure better blood glucose control. Raw or partially ripe fruits are preferable for people with diabetes due to their lower sugar content. A whole fruit is preferred over fruit juice as it gives more satiety because of its fibre content. Having a fruit with some nuts (fruit and nut combination) will ensure the sustained release of glucose and maintain normal levels of blood glucose. Fruits work best before playtime for kids with Type 1 diabetes.

Space out your fruits. Two fruit portions each providing approximately 15 g of carbohydrates can be consumed in a day. However, the recommendation for each individual depends on your blood glucose levels or any other medical condition that you have where fruits may need to be restricted. It is recommended that you speak to your doctor and dietitian to know the amount of fruit you can eat in a day.

Fruit Portions

1 Fruit portion

Apple	–	1 medium
Pear	–	1 medium
Guava	–	1 medium
Pomegranate	–	½ bowl
Orange	–	1 medium
Litchi	–	3–4 no. (small)
Papaya	–	1 bowl
Pineapple	–	3 slices
Mango	–	2 slices
Watermelon	–	1 bowl
Banana	–	1 elaichi banana/½ regular banana
Strawberries	–	5–6 no.
Cherries	–	10 no.
Chickoo/Sapota	–	1 small
Grapes	–	15 no.

Frequently Asked Question

Can people with diabetes tango to a mango?

When some people say that even if you have diabetes, you can eat a mango using social media as a medium of communication, all hell breaks loose and we have our patients with diabetes buying mangoes by the dozens and having it as mango juice, aamras and milkshakes. It is indeed a crazy time of the year for all dietitians and physicians managing the skyrocketing blood glucose levels of their patients.

So the question arises, if people with diabetes can consume mangoes or not. The good news is that, yes, of course a person with diabetes can consume mangoes, but they need to know how much and when to eat. They also need to know when not to eat it.

Mango is a nutritious fruit containing many essential nutrients and the bioactive compound mangiferin which has demonstrated to exert protective effects against degenerative diseases such as heart disease, cancer, obesity and diabetes. It also protects the body against damage associated with oxidative stress.

120 g (1/2 cup cubed) of the edible portion of mango (Mangifera indica L.) gives approximately 15 g of carbs. Mangoes score 51–60 on the glycemic index chart depending on the variety of mango one buys and the glycemic load is between 7–9. It is therefore a medium glycemic index and a low glycemic load fruit making it safe for people with diabetes to eat in portioned amounts.

To consume or not to consume depends on the level of physical activity, HbA1c, blood glucose control and variability. If the blood glucose levels are well controlled, it is advisable to eat the fruit in between meals and not with food like most people do. This will spike up the post-meal blood glucose levels. The best time to consume a mango is before an activity so that the blood glucose levels remain stable. Do not have it as a juice or as an aamras or milkshake. Consume fresh mangoes only during its season (end April and May) to reap the maximum health benefits. It is best to consult your doctor or a qualified dietitian to know how much and how often you can eat this fruit!

Nuts and Oilseeds

Despite being high in fat and calories, nuts and oilseeds are power-packed with nutrients and extremely beneficial to health. It is a myth that nuts have cholesterol. Nuts and oilseeds are plant food, and hence are naturally cholesterol-free.

Nuts and seeds are very low in carbohydrates, with good amounts of heart-healthy fats, fibre, and protein. This makes nuts an ideal choice for people with diabetes as well as for weight watchers. Studies have shown that people who ate a handful of nuts daily enjoyed a prolonged life and improved heart health. Nuts consumed before meals have also shown to help improve the post meal blood glucose levels. Walnut consumption has also shown to curb cravings for unhealthy foods.

Ensure you eat them in moderation as they are also a dense source of calories. Choose unsalted nuts to get its maximum nutrient benefits.

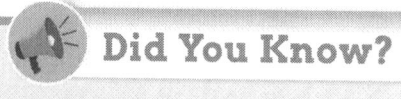

Did You Know?

100 calorie portion of nuts

Cashew nut – 12 no.

Almonds – 15 no.

Pistachios – 22 no.

Walnuts – 5 halves

Fats and Oils

These foods should be taken in limited amounts as they are rich sources of calories. It is not recommended that you go on a fat-free diet as fat is an essential nutrient and important for the absorption of several important fat-soluble nutrients like vitamin A, D, E and K and carotenoids.

It is advisable to limit saturated fat and trans-fats. Choose healthy oils (refer to the chapter on fats and oils). Go easy on the salad dressings, sugar-free ice creams, and any other commercially available sugar-free sweets as they have high amounts of invisible fat.

Fat enters your diet in various forms such as full-fat milk and milk products, high-fat salad dressings or on the addition of cream, butter, mayonnaise, cheese, to your food.

Remember, Moderation Is Key!

Real life example

Krutika (name changed) visited me for diet counselling; she had diabetes with high cholesterol and triglyceride levels. I suggested, "You need to cut down on refined and fatty foods." She said, "I do not eat fried food like puri, bhatura, samosa, batatawada at all. I always stay away from deep-fried foods".

She was happy that she was making wise choices, but later during the consultation she shared that she ate a salad with her meal (her salad was made of fresh vegetables with mayo dressing), she ate a vegetable sandwich for breakfast (She added mayo and butter to that too) and usually noodles or ready-to-eat meals at dinner due to lack of time. Though Krutika did not have deep-fried foods, her meals had a lot of fat added to it. Moreover her consumption of refined flour was also high. It is important to look at what goes on our plate. You may unknowingly be having unhealthy foods which can be detrimental to your health.

> What goes on our plate will show on our waist.

Vitamins and Minerals

Vitamins and minerals are micro-nutrients; though they are present in small quantities, they are vital to life and growth. They do not provide energy (calories) but are essential for most body functions and all tissues of the body. Prolonged shortage of any of these can lead to deficiency disorders as each of them has a specific role to play in the body's functioning.

Vitamins are destroyed during storing, cooking and processing. Hence, the focus should be on using the right cooking and storing methods. A balanced diet with a wide variety of foods should provide most of the important vitamins and minerals. The daily requirements vary for each vitamin and mineral.

A new research has shown a link between vitamin D and diabetes. Most Indians have low vitamin D levels. Vitamin D sources include fatty fish like tuna, mackerel, salmon, egg yolks and fortified dairy products. Other foods fortified with vitamin D are also available now. Exposure to sunlight (between 11 A.M. to 2.P.M.) is important for the activation of vitamin D.

Our Indian diet is well-balanced and supplements are not required under normal circumstances. Supplements should be taken only on your doctor's recommendation. Minerals must be correctly balanced in the body to work efficiently. Most of the minerals get destroyed during refining and processing.

Most People love palak paneer and it is always on the menu – be it at home or at buffets or at restaurants. Did you know that palak paneer is not the best food choice for calcium or iron as calcium and iron compete with each other for absorption in the body?

By and large, studies show that calcium when taken with iron-rich food inhibits the absorption of iron from food.

Therefore it is advisable for people who have iron deficiency and anaemia to avoid taking calcium-rich foods or calcium supplements with meals to ensure enhanced absorption of iron from meals.

Calcium supplements, when prescribed, must preferably be taken when going to bed. Iron supplements taken with Vit C (unsweetened lemon juice) enhances absorption of iron.

Avoid having tea immediately after meals as it hinders the iron absorption.

Regular consumption of alcohol can reduce the bioavailability of important nutrients like Vit A, Vit B1, B2, B6, B12, folate and zinc.

Certain drugs can also cause depletion of vitamins and minerals. For example, prolonged usage of the anti-diabetes drugs – metformin, can cause low vitamin B12 levels.

Regular consumption of antacids, laxatives, diuretics can cause several mineral and vitamin deficiencies.

Speak to your doctor and dietitian to know how to get the best from your food when taking different drugs.

A wide variety of foods, with emphasis on unrefined foods, will help prevent deficiencies. Important minerals include calcium, phosphorus, iron, sodium, potassium, iodine, magnesium, copper, chromium, selenium and zinc.

Women, teenage girls and pregnant women should increase the intake of foods rich in calcium. Children, adolescents and women of childbearing age should make sure to consume iron-rich foods like garden cress seeds, red amaranth, brown chana, bajra, dried dates and rajma.

 Frequently Asked Question

My blood reports suggest I am Vitamin D deficient, I have started taking Vitamin D supplements as my neighbour suggested. Is it alright to take it for long?

Vitamin D toxicity, also called hypervitaminosis D, is a rare but serious condition that occurs when you have excessive amounts of vitamin D in your body.

Vitamin D toxicity is usually caused by taking high doses of vitamin D supplements. Vitamin D toxicity cannot be caused by diet or sun exposure. That is because our body regulates the amount of vitamin D activated by sun exposure and even fortified foods don't contain large amounts of vitamin D.

The main consequence of vitamin D toxicity is a build-up of calcium in the blood (hypercalcaemia), which can cause nausea and vomiting, weakness, and frequent urination. Symptoms might progress to kidney problems such as the formation of calcium stones and high creatinine levels.

Taking 60,000 international units (IU) a day of vitamin D for several months has been shown to cause toxicity. Vitamin D supplements, in case of deficiency, should be taken only with the recommendation of the doctor for a specified time frame. Blood levels should be monitored while you are on vitamin D supplements.

It is important to consume a diet rich in magnesium (dark leafy greens, almonds, pumpkin seeds, chia seeds, flaxseeds and whole grains) to balance out the excess calcium in the blood.

As always, talk to your doctor before taking any vitamin and mineral supplements. Do not take it at the behest of unqualified people.

Water

The human body is about 60% water which is used in almost every bodily function. It is one of the most effective hydrating agents and the best part is that it is calorie-free. Most of us sitting in air-conditioned offices often forget to drink water. I tell my patients to fill a litre of water, keep it at their desk and finish it by noon and another litre by evening. You can also flavour your water by adding mint, lemon, cinnamon and ginger. This will ensure that you meet your minimum recommended intake of at least two litres of water/day. It is scientifically recommended that you drink 35-40 ml water/kg body weight per day (unless advised against doing so by your doctor).

Avoid sugary drinks, fruit juices and colas since these are high in sugar content and increase your blood sugar levels.

> It is crucial we revisit our lifestyle and adopt healthy practices to enjoy a better quality life. It is time to go back to traditional eating practices and incorporate more whole foods which are less processed and refined in our diet.
>
> As the saying goes "If you wish to enjoy a healthy and long life, do not eat what your grandmother would not recognize as food."

Real life journey shared by Utkarshini

I am Utkarshini and I am 26 years old. I have Type 1 diabetes since the past 21 years. Initially, when I was diagnosed I had good control of my blood glucose levels. As I started growing, I wanted to explore more and try new things, but I still gave priority to my studies and achieved a gold medal in B. Pharm.

I decided to go to Canada to pursue higher education. Once I went abroad for further studies, my schedules were busy as I was also working simultaneously. At the same time there was a lot of freedom to make my own decisions. I had to independently take the responsibility to choose or succumb to my urge to explore new things.

I was still on the traditional short-acting insulin and intermediate-acting dose then which means I had to have meals even when I was working or in the lab.

The country was new, so the food was very different and its effect on my blood glucose levels was really hitting hard. I met an educator there to understand the food that I could choose.

I started putting on weight and my blood glucose levels were just not under control. 4 years passed and I was still fighting to keep my blood glucose levels in the target range.

When I came back to India, my HbA1c was 10.3. I met my diabetologist to get his guidance to manage my blood glucose levels. He explained to me, "You need to match your food and insulin. There are a lot of lows and highs. Correction of lows leads to high blood glucose levels. Hence, you need to reduce your total dosage."

He switched me from my conventional insulin dose to fast-acting insulin dose before meals and long-acting insulin dose at bedtime. He suggested I meet a dietitian and get my meals planned with her.

I have been lucky to meet her at the right time in my life. She helped me plan my daily meals keeping my schedules in mind (I have an outdoor job). She gave me options of food that I liked. She, in fact, taught me how to choose the right food and the correct way of eating. She never gave me any rigid diet schedules and she never said NO for anything.

In three months, my insulin dose reduced from 45 to 34 units. My blood glucose level is in good control and my present HbA1c is 7.3 and above all I have lost 6 kg of weight without any extra effort. My total cholesterol has come down from 253 to 170, only by making changes in the meal plan.

I have learnt from her to make prudent choices on what to eat, how much to eat and what is the best time to enjoy a particular food. My body is now tuned in a manner that I feel full with 30–40 gm carbs, which is the recommended amount at each meal for me.

I would like to say that I had two phases in my life where I was a rebel in terms of diabetes as I was told "You can eat this" or "You cannot eat this."

But after I met my dietitian, my relationship with food has changed. **I feel getting the right education about the food that you eat is very important.** You need to learn the nuances of portion control and carbohydrate counting and your blood glucose levels will be managed automatically.

Key takeaways

- Healthy Food Plate with all nutrients is crucial for a healthy and fit body. Use food as your medicine.
- Focused dietary counselling will enable good meal planning.
- Portion control is important. Choose smaller plates and bowls.
- Quality and Quantity of food matters. Moderation is key.

CHAPTER 02
Are You in the Safe Zone? – Let's Find Out

As we are all aware, we are facing a tsunami of lifestyle diseases such as diabetes, hypertension, obesity, high cholesterol levels owing to today's faulty lifestyle – high consumption of simple sugars and refined foods, high stress levels, less moving and more sitting leading to obesity and increased fat in the body (adiposity)

Let's do the risk assessment for ourselves and our families and see if we are in the safe zone.

Are you in the ideal body weight zone?

Being overweight puts an individual at an increased risk of lifestyle diseases and diabetes related complications

- Ideal body weight = Ht. in cms –100(for Males)
- For eg. Male – 160 cm tall
- IBW = 160–100 = 60kg
- Ideal body weight = Ht. in cm –105(for Females)
- For eg. Female – 160 cm tall
- IBW = 160–105 = 55 kg
- \> 20% is considered to be overweight
- < 20% is considered to be underweight

Body Mass Index (BMI), a ratio of weight to height, is considered one of the measures for assessing an individual's overall health risk. It is defined as the weight in kilograms divided by the square of the height in meters (kg/m^2). Getting the BMI into a healthy range is important to reduce the risk of lifestyle disease and diabetes. As Indians are more predisposed to lifestyle diseases like diabetes, the suggested cut offs for BMI is 22.9 kg/m2 in Asian Indians as against 25kg/m2 in Caucasians

Body Mass Index (BMI (for Asian Indians):

BMI(kg/m2)	Classification
≤ 18.5	Underweight
18.6–22.9	Normal body weight
23–24.9	Overweight
≥ 25	Obese

If the BMI falls in the overweight or obese category, the individual is at a higher risk for various chronic lifestyle diseases such as diabetes, hypertension, heart disease, etc.

Waist Circumference:

Body fat around the waist (central obesity) is a common culprit of lifestyle diseases. Remember "Longer the belt shorter is the lifespan". You are more predisposed to lifestyle diseases if your waistline is more than 35 inches (90 cm) if you are a man or 32 inches (80 cm) if you are a woman.

Waist to height ratio:

Since an individual cannot change his height, he should take special care to keep his weight and in particular, waist (abdominal girth) in the healthy range

The **Waist to height ratio (WHtR)** gives a more accurate assessment of health since the most dangerous place to carry weight is in the abdomen. Fat in the abdomen, which is associated with a larger waist, is metabolically active and produces various hormones that can cause harmful effects, such as diabetes, elevated blood pressure and altered lipid (blood fat) levels.

- Waist in inches or cm/height in inches or cm × 100 = WHtR
- eg: a Male with a 32 inch waist who is 5'10" (70 inches) would divide 32 by 70, to get a WHtR of 45.7 percent.

ARE YOU IN THE SAFE ZONE?

Average height
5ft 10in (70in) — 35 in
5ft 6in (66in) — 35 in

Your waist should be half your height

WOMEN - Waist to Height Ratios
Under 35: Abnormally Thin
35 to 42: Extremely Slim
42 to 49: Healthy
49 to 54: Overweight
54 to 58: Seriously Overweight
Over 58: Extremely Obese

MEN - Waist to Height Ratios
Under 35: Abnormally Thin
35 to 43: Extremely Slim
43 to 53: Healthy
53 to 58: Overweight
58 to 63: Seriously Overweight
Over 63: Extremely Obese

Indians are known to be **thin fat people**. We appear slim but have excess body fat with more concentration of fat in the abdominal area (visceral fat) putting us at an increased risk of lifestyle diseases. We usually have lower levels of muscle mass. Muscle is metabolically more active than fat. Those having higher body fat levels have a sluggish metabolism making it more difficult for them to lose weight. It is important to do your body composition to know where you stand and can take corrective action to lower your risk.

Get your ABCs checked regularly – A1c Blood pressure, and Blood cholesterol. By keeping your ABC's under control, you can lower your risk of diabetes complications. Recommended targets are HbA1c of < 7%, blood pressure < 140/80 mmHg, LDL (bad cholesterol) < 100mg/dl, HDL (good cholesterol) > 40mg/dl for men and > 50 mg/dl for females, triglycerides < 150mg/dl. Talk to your doctor about setting individualistic targets for you.

Take the Indian Diabetes Risk Score developed by Dr. V. Mohan and team to know yours and your families risk of developing diabetes.

Indian Diabetes Risk Score (IDRS)

Parameter	Score	Your Score
Age		
< 35 years	0	
35–49 years	20	
≥ 50 years	30	
Waist circumference		
Waist < 80cm – Females, < 90cm – Males	0	
Waist ≥ 80–89cm – Females, ≥ 90–99cm – Males	10	
Waist ≥ 90cm – Females, ≥ 100cm – Males	20	
Physical activity		
Regular vigorous exercise or strenuous (manual) activities at home/work	0	
Regular moderate exercise or moderate physical activity at home/work	10	
Regular mild exercise or mild physical activity at home/work	20	
No exercise and/or sedentary activities at home/work	30	
Family history		

No history of diabetes in parents	0
One parent is having diabetes	10
Both parents are having diabetes	20
Total	

Risk	Score
Low risk	< 30
Moderate risk	30–60
High risk	≥ 60

Real life example

A 42-year-old lady, Saba (name changed) did her annual health check-up recently. Her HbA1c was 6%, fasting blood glucose levels were 101 mg/dl and post meal blood glucose levels was 93 mg/dl. She was obese with a BMI of more than 30 kg/m2 and had abdominal obesity (waist circumference > 36 inches or 91 cm). Her waist to height ratio was 60. There was no physical activity and she often ate unhealthy especially when stressed or bored.

She was very happy to see that her post meal blood glucose levels were lesser than her fasting blood glucose level. She thought that this gave her the liberty to eat sweets and cakes. She was referred to us for weight loss by her friend who was our patient. At the beginning of the consultation, I discussed the reports in detail with her. Her HbA1c indicated that she had pre-diabetes (HbA1c-6 %). Her post meal blood glucose levels being lower than her fasting blood glucose levels was infact a matter of concern as it indicated hyperinsulinemia (increased insulin levels) due to insulin resistance (increased fat making insulin action ineffective). This was a sign that she had an increased risk of developing diabetes in the near future.

She had most of the risk factors for developing diabetes, she was obese with a waist circumference more than the desired range.

Her parents had diabetes and hypertension. She was physically inactive and wasn't careful about her food.

She promised to immediately take action and work on changing her lifestyle. We planned a diet and exercise plan which helped her lose weight and reduce inches especially on the waist. She started feeling better and her HbA1c reduced to 5.5% in the next four months. Her fasting blood glucose levels was below 90 mg/dl and post meal blood glucose levels were also in the desired range. She was happy and thankful to her friend who referred her to us for guidance at the right time.

Sit less, Move more, Eat right, Eat Light, Stress less, Sleep well and make efforts to increase physical activity through the day.

CHAPTER 03 Proteins

Proteins are specialised nutrients and the building materials of the body responsible for growth, maintenance, immunity and energy. A survey titled 'Protein Consumption in Diet of Adult Indians (PRODIGY)' indicates that **9 out of 10** people consume inadequate amounts of protein in India. Statistics revealed that 93% of the Indian population is unaware of the ideal protein requirement per day with pregnant ladies on the top (97%), followed by lactating mothers (96%) and adolescents (95%). According to The Indian Market Research Bureau's 2017 report, **protein deficiency among Indians stands at more than 80 percent,** measured against the recommended 60 g per day.

In today's era of social media diets and fad diets where most of the times, there is a complete exclusion of one or more food groups, protein deficiency is becoming more and more common and a matter of concern today.

Also when people don't eat carbs and eat only protein, the protein is used as a source of energy and not spared for bodybuilding and other important functions.

Below is the diet recall of Mrs. Janaki (name changed), a 49-year-old, South Indian female, vegetarian, weighing 58 kg, 5 feet 5 inches (165 cm) tall.

Meal/Timings	Menu	Household measures	Protein(g/day)
Early morning	Tea	1 cup	1.6
Breakfast	Upma/Poha	1 soup bowl	5
	Milk	1 cup	4.5
Mid morning	Fruit	1 no.	-
Lunch	Rice	1 soup bowl	3
	Vegetable curry	1 soup bowl	-
	Dal	1 dessert bowl(thin)	3.5
Evening	Tea	1 cup	1.6
	Puffed rice	1 soup bowl	1.4
Dinner	Rice	1 soup bowl	3
	Vegetable	1 soup bowl	0.5
	Tomato Rassam	1 soup bowl (thin)	0.2
	Total		24.3

Present body weight = 58Kgs Height – 165 cm, Her ideal body weight is 60 kg.

Total Protein intake – 24.3 g/day = 0.4 g/Kg present body weight.,

On an average, an apparently healthy individual needs 0.8–1.0 g of protein per kg of ideal body weight.

The protein requirements may vary depending on several factors such as physical activity, age, medical conditions such as kidney disease etc.

For Mrs. Janaki's ideal body weight of 60 kg, she must consume at least 48–60 g of protein.

Consuming lesser protein over time can lead to loss of muscle mass (sarcopenia), lowered metabolism, low energy levels, reduced immunity, poor quality hair, weak and brittle nails etc.

Adding protein to meals not only helps blunt the blood glucose spike post-meals but also gives a feeling of satiety. Post-workout snack must always be a good quality protein source.

Sources of protein include milk and milk products, dals, sprouts, pulses (chana, moong, matki, rajma), soyabean, egg, meat, fish, chicken and nuts.

For vegetarians who find it difficult to meet your protein intake, milk, yoghurt, buttermilk, whey water, hung curd, low-fat paneer, cheese, soyabean and tofu are excellent sources of high-quality protein and must be included in your meal plan.

As discussed in the earlier chapter, combining cereals with pulses helps to improve the protein quality of the meal (e.g.: Khichdi, idli, dosa)

Meeting your protein requirements

Source	Amount	Protein Content
Milk (Cow's)	150 ml (1 cup)	4.8 g
Curd	100 g (5½ tbsp*)	3.2 g
Paneer (cottage cheese)	50 g	9.4 g
Cheese	25 g (1 cheese cube)	5.8 g
Greek yogurt	100 g	8.2 g
Pulses (moong, rajma, chana)	30 g (1 fistful)	7.0 g
Soybean	25 g	8.8 g
Soya chunks (raw)	30 g (¾ cup)	15 g
Soy paneer (tofu)	100 g	7.7 g
Egg	1 whole/2 whites	6.5 g
Chicken/Fish/Mutton	100 g	18–20 g

*tbsp (Tablespoon)

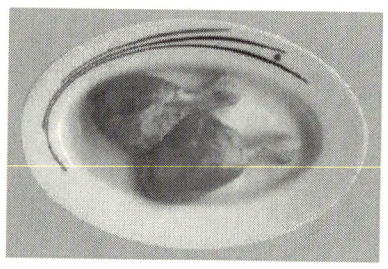 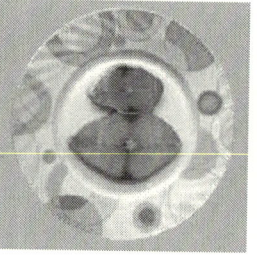 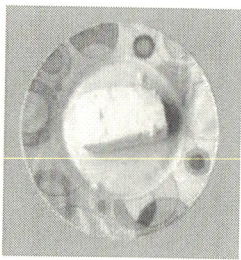

100 g Chicken   **100 g Fish**   **50 g Paneer (cottage cheese)**

Choose low-fat protein sources like lean meat, sprouts, egg whites, low-fat milk. Ensure that a protein source from the list given above is always there at lunch and dinner.

Ways to include protein in the diet at breakfast are:

- Pessarattu (moong dal)/mix dal dosa/Besan (chickpea flour) dosa/chilla
- Paniyarams made from pulses
- Spanish omelette/boiled egg/poached egg/egg omelette
- Idli with sambar
- Pulse moong (green gram), moth beans (matki), kidney beans (rajma), Chickpea (kabuli chana)/soya tikkis
- Sattu (chickpea flour) drink/parathas
- Add a glass of buttermilk or curd to the breakfast of poha, upma
- Reduce on the quantity of poha/upma and add an egg or a bowl of sprouts or curd

Choose from the following options for your mid-meal snacks-

Chana-peanut combination, a dal chilla, dal paniyarams, chana chaat, eggs, paneer tikka, scrambled tofu, hung curd, plain yogurt, soynuts, buttermilk, hummus/hung curd dip with carrot cucumber sticks, sattu drink.

It is not advisable to have excess amounts of protein as it causes a load on your kidneys. Your dietitian will help you understand the amount of protein you need to consume depending on your height, weight, physical activity and blood reports.

Effect of protein on blood glucose levels

Protein eaten in small portions has little effect on blood glucose levels. But if you eat large amounts of protein in a meal (3 servings of protein = 3 × 7 g of protein/serving = 21 g of protein)*, it may delay the absorption of carbohydrates and will cause the blood glucose levels to increase after a few hours of the meal. Frequent blood glucose monitoring in such situations is recommended.

If you eat more than 120 g fish/chicken (thicker than a deck of cards and larger than the palm of your hand).

In Summary

- *Ensure you meet your protein requirement of 0.8–1 g protein/kg ideal body weight (for people with no other medical condition)*
- *Include protein in every meal to blunt the post-meal glucose levels*
- *Include good quality protein or a cereal pulse combination which makes it a complete protein*
- *Opt for a protein-rich meal at mid-meals to help achieve satiety and maintain the blood glucose levels in the desired range.*

CHAPTER 04 Fats and Oils

Fats have earned a bad reputation over the years. Many people on a weight loss diet go off fat completely in the pursuit of quick and drastic weight loss. However one should not completely avoid fat in the diet as it is essential to the body.

Fats play a vital role in

1. promoting the absorption of the four fat-soluble vitamins (A, D, E and K) and are required for the synthesis of hormones
2. providing a feeling of fullness and satisfaction
3. increasing palatability
4. preserving the food longer

All fats are high in calories. Unlike carbs and protein that give 4 kcal per gram, each gram of fat gives 9 kcal. When taken in excess amounts, fats increase the risk of obesity, heart disease, stroke and cancer.

Real Life Example

Priyanka (name changed) had diabetes and she came to me as her doctor had advised her to lose weight and manage her blood glucose levels well. She is an AVP – Marketing in an MNC and her job involves long working hours. During consultation, she said that she lived with her husband and cooked food herself. She said, "I cook and eat everything that is healthy and use oil sparingly. I am very particular and cook food in extra virgin olive oil only and use only 1 litre of oil per month." During the conversation, I found out that though her overall fat consumption was moderate, she frequently travelled for work and was compelled to eat out often. Though her quantity of oil consumption at home was acceptable, there were two things hidden in it.

Firstly, the amount of oil and fat used in the food cooked outside is much more than the food cooked at home. This fat consumption when added to her regular intake was much more than the desired limits.

Secondly, using olive oil = good health is a myth. All oils have the same calories and should be used judiciously. Whether you use olive oil, or rice bran oil or sunflower oil or any other oil, the oil intake for every individual remains the same. Additionally, extra virgin olive oil has a low smoking point hence is not very adaptable for Indian cuisine which is generally cooked using high heat.

I designed a meal plan and suggested healthy options while eating out. She followed the instructions and she started losing weight easily.

If you look minutely at your daily food intake, you will notice that there is a lot of hidden fat consumed in your daily meal.

There are some families who still follow the traditional way of cooking using liberal oil/ghee in their food. It is healthy to eat traditional home-cooked food but it is important to keep a check on the amount of oil used.

Any fat or oil you eat (healthy or unhealthy) is a dense source of calories. Remember, we are not as active as our ancestors were, hence we do not burn as many calories as they did.

The recommendation for fat intake would differ depending on your health goals and activity levels. On average, an individual recommendation of oil is 3 level tsp or 1 level tablespoon/day which works out to ½ a litre per month. However this depends on your activity level and would differ for each individual.

Fats Can Be Categorised as

a) Healthy Fats - Unsaturated Fats

They are classified as monounsaturated (MUFA) and polyunsaturated fats (PUFA). It is recommended that you get 10–15% of your fat calories from monounsaturated fatty acids. The intake of polyunsaturated fatty acids should be 8–10% of energy intake. They are essential because they cannot be synthesized by the body and have to be obtained from dietary sources. There are two families of PUFA that are essential: Omega-6 and Omega-3.

Omega-6 fatty acids (n-6) support the heart, improve immunity, and nervous system function. Omega-3 fatty acids (n-3) on the other hand prevents clogging of the arteries, protects against diseases like arthritis and colitis, reduces your risk of cancer and Alzheimer's. Eating fatty fish, prepared in a healthy manner, 2 to 3 times a week gives protection to the heart.

Healthy Fats

Unsaturated fats found in many vegetable oils and seeds do not raise blood cholesterol levels and have a protective effect on the heart. Even though they are considered healthy, healthy fats are still high in calories. They can be made part of a healthy diet, as long as you do not exceed your total fat allowance.

Monounsaturated Fats (MUFA)	Polyunsaturated Fats (PUFA): Omega-6	Polyunsaturated Fats (PUFA): Omega-3
Decreases LDL (bad) Cholesterol	Decreases LDL (bad) cholesterol and improves insulin action.	Reduces Triglycerides and stickiness in blood
Sources: Olive oil, Groundnut oil, Canola oil, Rice Bran Oil, Nuts, Olives, Sesame seeds, Avocado,	**Sources:** Safflower, Sunflower, Cottonseed, Corn, Soyabean oil, Groundnut, Rice bran and Sesame oil.	**Sources:** Soyabean, Canola and Mustard oils, pulses like Black Gram (kala chana), Kidney beans (rajmah) and Cowpea (lobia), Mustard and Fenugreek seeds and green leafy vegetables, fish like Mackerel, Sardines, Chia seeds, Flaxseeds, Walnuts, Tuna and Salmon.

Different types of olive oil: Which one to buy?

Using olive oil for cooking these days has become a trend. It is considered a much healthier oil. Olive oil is a wonderful source of monounsaturated fatty acid and antioxidants. When you are in a supermarket, you see different types of olive oils on the shelf for different prices – Extra Virgin Olive Oil, Virgin Olive Oil, Refined Olive Oil, Pomace Olive Oil and are left confused as to which one to buy.

So what's the difference and which one is best for you and your family?

EXTRA VIRGIN OLIVE OIL

- **Highest quality, is produced by cold pressing freshly picked olives**
- **Richest in antioxidant**
- **Greenish golden to bright green in colour, has a strong aroma and taste**
- **Unstable when exposed to heat, high heat cooking destroys its nutritional value**
- *Extra virgin olive oil is best used in salads and dips*

VIRGIN OLIVE OIL

- Virgin olive is good for cooking purpose, mainly for sautéing and baking
- Can be used in salads as well
- *Virgin olive oil is good for body and hair massage too*

REFINED OLIVE OIL

- It is obtained by refining virgin olive oil
- It is made for bulk consumption and is comparatively cheaper
- It does not have the characteristic flavour, taste or aroma of pure olive oil
- *Refined olive oil is suitable for cooking. Avoid its use in salads*

OLIVE POMACE OIL

- When all the oil and water is extracted from olives, there is still some oil residue left that can be extracted from olive pomace
- This olive pomace oil is then blended with virgin olive oil to impart some of the benefits of olive oil
- *Olive Pomace oil is good for high heat cooking*

LITE OLIVE OIL or LIGHT OLIVE OIL

- Generally, people get confused with the term "lite" thinking it means low in calories, however that's not true when it comes to oils
- Lite olive oil is a very low-grade version of olive oil but has the same amount of calories. However, it is low in its nutritional value, taste and aroma
- *Light or Lite olive oil is suitable for cooking and baking*

Real Life Example

Ritvik (name changed) was overweight and had diabetes with high cholesterol levels. He felt weak and tired easily. Along with the medications, the doctor advised him to make changes in his diet and start an exercise routine of walking for at least 20–25 minutes each day.

He visited my clinic for diet consultation. During his assessment and taking a detailed diet recall, he mentioned that they were a family of four using 10 litres of oil (including ghee) in a month. The maharaj cooked their meals and was very liberal with his usage of oil and ghee. Ritvik ate 2 Gujarati bhakris and 1 soup bowl of rice in his lunch daily. His maharaj added at least 2 spoons of oil while kneading the bhakri dough. He ate home-cooked food on most days with dinner being snack items like ragda pattice, panipuri, thepla chunda, sandwich, dosa etc. Evening snack was khakra with farsan daily.

They also consumed fried items on a regular basis. I made changes in his eating pattern. I asked him to get his cook and explained to the cook the right ways of cooking. I asked him to remove aside the daily allowance of oil for the day and make food only in that much oil. I also educated him on the cooking methods and utensils he could use to minimize oil consumption. I asked Ritvik to eat a handful of unsalted nuts like almonds and pistas instead of the khakra with farsan.

Ritvik started losing weight and monitored his blood glucose regularly. He started feeling fresh and energetic. His HbA1c and his cholesterol levels also showed an improvement in three months.

Fats are important for our bodies, but they should be used judiciously. **Remember, no fat or oil is "totally safe" and cannot be consumed in unlimited quantities.**

Most of us are slaves to our tongues and enjoy tasty food. And if we have cooks, the matter just gets worse. They have no control over the oil usage; their only goal is to serve you tasty food.

b) Unhealthy fats - Saturated fats and Trans-fat

Unhealthy fats increase your chances of heart disease and stroke. Unhealthy fats like saturated fat and trans-fat increase your blood cholesterol and can cause a build-up of materials that can clog your blood vessels. The blood supply to your heart can be blocked, leading to a heart attack. A blockage in the blood vessels going to your brain can result in paralysis or stroke. Saturated fat can cause a decrease in beta cells that produce insulin and are thus associated with several metabolic diseases including Type 2 DM.

Many studies have shown that trans-fats tend to raise LDL (bad) cholesterol and lower HDL (good) cholesterol.

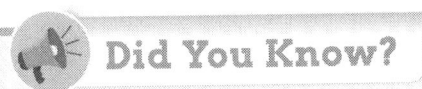

Did You Know?

"According to the well-known Framingham Heart Study, eating just one extra tablespoon of margarine increased a man's chances of heart attack by 10%."

Recent studies have suggested that trans-fats may also increase your chances of infertility, getting some kinds of cancer, including breast cancer and colon cancer. It greatly increases a pregnant woman's risk of preeclampsia and may harm her foetus. For people with diabetes, trans-fats lower your body's response to insulin. World Health Organisation (WHO) and the FSSAI want to cut down trans-fats to zero by 2023.

Ensure that you read the food label and look for trans-fats before buying any product.

Dietary Cholesterol

Cholesterol synthesis takes place in the liver and some of it comes from the food that we eat.

This is one of my favourites. I often hear people say this, "I use only 'cholesterol-free oil'; hence I can be assured of good health."

Most overweight people try to justify excess oil consumption by saying that they are using cholesterol-free oil. Do not fall prey to these claims. It is a great marketing gimmick by the manufacturers to boost sales. Remember, all vegetarian foods are cholesterol-free including the very controversial cashew nut and coconut.

 Frequently Asked Question

To yolk or not to yolk?

This is a question often asked by my patients.

In the past, eggs received a lot of bad publicity due to the high cholesterol content in the egg yolk. Egg yolk has always been considered a villain in the past with healthcare professionals asking people to avoid the yolk and eat only the white of the egg.

In 2015, the Dietary Guidelines for Americans removed the recommendations of setting a limit to the maximum intake of 300 mg/day cholesterol as extensive research did not show evidence to support a role of dietary cholesterol in the development of heart disease.

A recent study published in the Journal of the American Medical Association in 2019 found that each additional 300 mg of dietary cholesterol consumed per day was significantly associated with a higher risk of heart disease. This left everyone confused whether to recommend a whole egg with yolk or not.

An egg is a power-packed food with many vital nutrients. It is a high biological value protein, only source of albumin, the yolk has the fat-soluble vitamins – Vit D and Vit A, Zinc, choline and biotin which are essential nutrients for health. The cholesterol in one whole egg is only 183 mg which is well within the recommendation. Indians eat a lot of carbs and unhealthy fats especially in the evening when hunger pangs strike. A whole egg with two whites will not only give 12 grams of good quality protein but also has zero carbs. A healthy swap for the biscuits, samosas, vadas which are high in carbs and unhealthy fats. An egg at breakfast improves satiety and reduces the post-meal blood glucose spikes.

> Studies have shown that daily consumption of one large egg may reduce the risk of diabetes without having any adverse effects on cholesterol levels in individuals with pre-diabetes and Type 2 diabetes. Ensure that the egg is cooked in a healthy manner and not with too much oil or butter.

Unhealthy Fats

They raise blood cholesterol levels and put you at an increased risk for obesity, diabetes, heart disease and cancer.

Saturated Fats	Trans-fats	Dietary Cholesterol
Restrict foods with too much saturated fat as they raise 'bad cholesterol' levels in your blood. Saturated fats should be restricted to < 10% of the total energy and < 6–7% in those with deranged lipid profile	Eat foods with as little trans-fat as possible (less than 1% of total energy). Trans-fats should be preferably totally avoided.	Restrict the dietary cholesterol intake to less than 300 mg/day. There should be a restricted intake of foods which have cholesterol.
Sources: Butter, cheese, ghee, whole milk and cream, egg yolks, lard and skin of poultry, red meat and processed meat like sausages, ham and bacon, coconut oil, cocoa butter and palm kernel oils.	**Sources:** Bakery products, margarine, vanaspati/dalda, ready-to-eat (processed) foods, deep-fried foods like samosas, bhajias, French fries, chips, sweets like jalebis, gulab jamuns, etc.	**Sources:** Milk and milk products, butter, ghee, egg yolks, liver, brain and other organ meats, red meat and poultry.

> Look for words such as "shortening", "partially hydrogenated vegetable oil" or "hydrogenated vegetable oil" in the ingredients. These words are clues that the food contains trans-fat.

Did You Know?

Roasting flaxseeds on high flame increases the amount of trans-fats.

A common practice followed here is that we roast it on a high flame (mostly on a tawa after roasting chapatis). The right way is to grind it and consume it immediately. In case it is not possible to freshly grind due to paucity of time, lightly roast flaxseed (to prevent it from getting rancid) on a pan and store in an airtight container in the refrigerator and consume it.

Nowadays, you get cold pressed ground flaxseed powder or oil in the supermarkets or even on e-commerce websites.

Did You Know?

Did you know that shallow frying soaks in more oil than deep frying?

There is a common misconception that deep frying takes in more oil than shallow frying. In fact, on the contrary, it is the other way around. In deep frying, the oil is hot (usually 300–375 degree F). This heat causes the water in the food to turn to steam, creating pressure, which keeps the oil from penetrating into the food. On the other hand, when you shallow fry the food, the top of the food is outside the oil and so is cooler than the part of the food which is in the oil. If the temperature drops below 212 degrees F, you do not have the steam pressure keeping the oil out, therefore causing the food to soak up more oil. Thus in most cases, shallow frying takes in more oil than deep frying for e.g.: If you eat a paratha at a dhaba in North India which is shallow fried on a tava, you will be surprised to know that it has more fat than a deep-fried puri.

A healthy cooking tip

You do not need to invest in expensive equipment for oil-free cooking. You can now enjoy your pakodas, vadas and muffins without guilt by using paniyaram makers that require less oil for cooking.

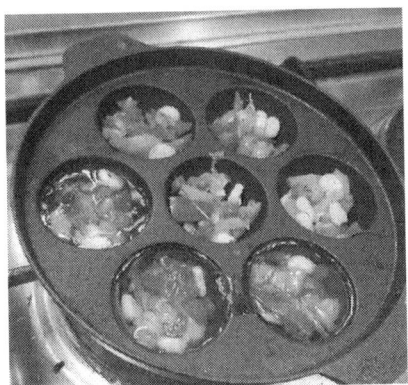

Paniyaram Maker

Cooking Sprays and Silicon Brushes

Cooking sprays are easily available in the market today and can be considered as a good option for low-fat cooking instead of using butter, oil or shortening. It can be sprayed on the pan, baking or microwave dish.

You can also use a silicon brush available easily in the market to grease dishes before cooking.

Frying and Reheating of Oils

For frying, use oils which have more stability and a high smoke point. The common practice of repeatedly using the oil for frying is hazardous as they generate free radicals and form a carcinogenic compound called acryl amide and trans-fats that are harmful to the health. On reheating, the viscosity of oil increases and becomes darker in colour and turns rancid. Therefore it is advisable not to reheat oils. The oil once used for frying can be used for cooking e.g. to give tadka to the dal.

One can reduce the risk of heart disease by eating right and exercising regularly. A plant-based diet has shown greater benefits in lowering the risk of heart disease.

> Keep this in mind when choosing oils. Oil should be trans-fat free and low in saturated fats.
>
> Use of mixed (blend) oils or alternating of oils is recommended to enjoy maximum health benefits.

Choice of Cooking Oils

No oil is fully saturated or unsaturated and can meet the ratio of SFA: PUFA: MUFA and n-6:n-3 as desired. Choose a combination of oils which maintains a balance to provide all the essential nutrients. For ensuring this appropriate balance of fatty acids in cereal-based diets (cereals are a good source of Omega-6 fatty acid), it is necessary to increase the Omega-3 fatty acid intake and reduce the quantity of Omega-6 fatty acid obtained from the cooking oil. To get good fats from the diet, it is advisable to consume more than one type of vegetable oils.

National Institute of Nutrition recommends a blend of two or more vegetable oils to be used in daily cooking. Commercially blended oils must be used and different oils must not be mixed at home as stability of oils is maintained in commercially blended oils.

> Recommendations from the National Institute of Nutrition to maintain the desired Omega-6 to Omega-3 ratios are as below.
>
> Groundnut/Sesame/Rice bran + Mustard oil
>
> Groundnut/Sesame/Rice bran + Soybean oil

Use healthy cooking options like grilling, broiling, baking, steaming, sautéing and stir frying.

Speak to your dietitian and find out which is the best oil for you and your family.

Oils must be rotated, different types of oils and not the same oil of different brands.

The humble coconut oil: Should you consider?

Coconut oil, once used widely by our grandparents, especially in south India was until the recent past, considered a villain responsible for heart disease. It is now making a comeback and is being lauded for its various health benefits.

There are many documented studies showing the positive influence of coconut oil seen in patients with Alzheimer's.

Similar effects have been noticed in conditions like hypothyroidism, abdominal obesity and hormonal imbalance. Coconut oil works efficiently in treating these abnormalities; although researchers are yet to establish these facts.

You can enjoy your authentic south Indian cuisine by cooking it in a moderate amount of coconut oil (within the daily budget of saturated fat) and gain health benefits.

Ghee: Good or Bad

Desi ghee or clarified butter that we have seen being churned with much love by our grandmothers has earned a bad reputation over the years and is often considered a villain. Many people on a weight loss diet go off ghee completely in the pursuit of a quick and drastic weight loss.

Yes, there have been concerns about the possibility of ghee contributing to an increased risk of heart disease since it contains a high percentage of saturated fatty acids, leading to increased production of cholesterol. The American Heart Association recommends limiting the consumption of saturated fats to less than 5 to 6% of the total day's calories to reduce the risk of heart disease.

You will be happy to know that desi ghee or clarified butter, often blamed for obesity and heart disease, is not that bad after all. Studies have shown that 5 and 10% ghee-supplemented diets fed for 2 weeks to 2 months did not have any significant effect on blood cholesterol and triglyceride levels.

Ghee obtained from grass-fed cows is a rich natural source of the nutrient Conjugated Linoleic Acid (CLA). CLA has many health benefits such as combating cancer, asthma, improving insulin action, improving blood pressure levels, and boosting immunity. Research has shown that CLA has been beneficial in lowering body fat and increasing lean body mass and thus improving metabolism. It is also said to be good for the nerves and brain besides nourishing the eyes, hair and skin.

Deep Frying in ghee is not recommended as it leads to the formation of products which are harmful to the heart. Ghee can be used to give vaghar/tadka (on low flame) or applied on chapattis.

This however does not mean you can go ahead with a liberal amount of ghee in your diet.

One must ensure that the intake of total fat (including ghee and coconut oil) should not exceed the prescribed limit of fat consumption. **For example:** If the budget of oil is 3 tsp, 1 tsp can be ghee or coconut oil which is the budget of saturated fat/day).

One word of advice here is to preferably use homemade ghee or buy an authentic brand of ghee.

> Remember, MODERATION IS KEY

Beware of hidden fats in packaged foods.

The oil used in most packaged foods (including dry farsan and biscuits) and commercially sold snacks is saturated fat as it is odourless and inexpensive compared to other oils. Therefore, it is advised to read the ingredients on the labels and eat as much less out of packets as possible. It is recommended that you make snacks at home as you know the quality of oil you are using.

- Right storage of oil is very important.
- The bottle containing oil should have a tight-fitting cap or else it will oxidise and deteriorate faster.
- A dark coloured bottle must be used as sunlight degrades the quality of the oil.
- Excessive heat or prolonged exposure to light will speed up flavour deterioration. Keep away from light and heat in a dry and dark place.
- Keep oil in clean and dry bottle as exposure to moisture will subject oil to oxidation, eventually leading to rancidity.
- Filter particles once oil is used for frying.

Which one to use – Refined, filtered or Kachchi ghani?

Refined oils are generally treated with chemicals to rid the oil of the impurities, odour and give it a more clear appearance. Most oils sold in the market are refined oils. They are more stable and can be stored for up to twelve months.

Filtered oils are oils filtered through strainers or other equipment's to remove the solid particles and contaminants from the oil but no chemicals are used in the process. They are generally dark and cloudy in appearance and have a peculiar seed smell from which they are extracted

Kachchi ghani refers to cold press extraction process for taking out oil from seeds. Traditionally, oil from seeds were extracted in kohlus (a wooden cold press used with the help of a bullock). In this process, seeds are crushed at a low temperature so natural properties, antioxidants and essential oils are retained in the oil. They are not very stable and cannot be stored for long. Please check the manufacturing date of the oil when buying as the oil gets oxidised on keeping on the shelf of a supermarket for long. Food safety may be a concern with these oils.

Effect of Fat on Blood Glucose Levels

Fat in small amounts has a minimal effect on blood glucose levels. However, if fat is present in high amounts, it can slow down the absorption of glucose from the meal. The best example is that of ice cream. You can test this on yourself. If you eat an ice cream and test blood glucose after two hours, the chances are that you will not see a spike in blood glucose levels, however if you test after a few hours, blood glucose levels may be higher. Hence, monitoring in case of a high-fat meal needs to be done for up to 4–6 hours after consuming the meal.

Similarly when you eat pizza, cheese, which is used liberally while preparing pizza, has high-fat content. When you test blood glucose after two hours, the chances are that you will not see a spike in blood glucose levels, however if you test after a few hours, blood glucose levels may be higher. In fact blood glucose levels remain high for many hours after eating pizza.

High-fat food may not show an immediate effect on your blood glucose levels but will definitely work on your weight and waist level. Being overweight or having a larger waist line is not good for your blood glucose levels in the long run.

In Summary

- *Focus on both the quality and quantity of oil*
- *Keep added fat to the minimum (3 level teaspoons/day or 1 level tablespoon/day)*
- *Consult a qualified dietitian to know the type and amount of oil recommended for you to use*
- *Rotate oils or use commercially available blended oils to acquire a balance of fatty acids in the diet*
- *Avoid trans-fat foods*
- *Ensure proper storage and use of oil*
- *Avoid refrying or reusing of oil*

CHAPTER 05: The Carb Story

The Good and Bad Carbs

In recent times, carbohydrates, also known as 'carbs' have earned a bad reputation. From bringing about a spike in your blood glucose levels to increasing weight and much more, carbs are being blamed for being your foe rather than your friend.

I have come across people who ask questions like; will a carb-free diet help me improve my blood glucose levels or reverse diabetes? Will a carb-free diet help me lose weight?

I ask them is it sustainable? Can you avoid carbs for life? The answer is usually NO!

My advice to them is to moderate the carb intake rather than cutting off carbs completely from the diet. This is not only sustainable but helps prevent nutrient deficiencies and complications arising out of it in the long run.

Are you aware of the relationship between carbs and your blood glucose levels?

When you eat carb-containing foods, they are broken down into glucose immediately which enters your bloodstream. Blood glucose levels begin to rise fifteen minutes after eating carbohydrates and most of it is broken down into glucose within the first two hours of eating.

That is the reason carbs are known to raise your blood glucose levels faster than any other nutrient and have the maximum influence on blood glucose. The rise in blood glucose levels depends on the amount and the type of carbohydrate (complex, simple, refined) you eat.

The hormone insulin helps the cells in your body to take up glucose and use it for providing energy to the body. People with diabetes have a deficiency of insulin or insulin is not utilized effectively, resulting in high blood glucose levels. It is important for people with diabetes to understand which foods contain carbohydrate and how to use them in meal planning to their advantage.

For people with Type 1 Diabetes, the more carbohydrates you eat, the more insulin you will need. Therefore carbohydrate counting is absolutely necessary and the key to maintaining tight control over your blood glucose levels in people with Type 1 Diabetes.

> Just because you're going to count carbohydrates does not mean you can't eat them! In fact, if you eat a well-balanced diet, half the calories you eat (50%) will come from carbohydrates.

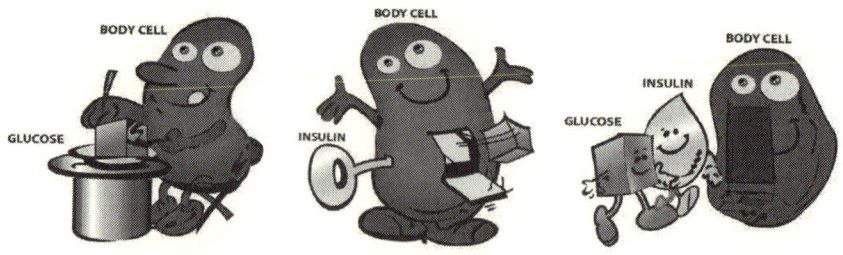

Just like petrol is the fuel to the car but the driver knows which petrol is good for the engine to work better, similarly it is important for you to know the good and bad carbs and what they do to your body.

CARBOHYDRATES

GOOD CARBOHYDRATES

BAD CARBOHYDRATES

COMPLEX CARBS

They are packed with fiber, vitamins and minerals. The body takes longer and has to work harder to break down these foods into energy. Include foods rich in complex carbohydrates as they give you sustained energy and keep you full longer and active throughout the day. Sources: Whole grain cereals – unpolished rice, whole wheat, oats, broken wheat (daliya), barley, buckwheat, millets- (jowar, bajra ,ragi (nachni), whole pulses and sprouts - soybeans, root vegetables, etc.

SIMPLE CARBS

They are digested quickly by the body. When taken in small amounts, they give your body an immediate energy boost. Best to correct a hypoglycemic event.

REFINED CARBS

The body processes refined carbohydrates quickly making your blood sugar rise and fall rapidly. The higher the food is in refined sugar, the worse it is for you as it offers very little nutritional value to your body.

Sources: Polished rice, white bread, white pasta, maida /refined flour and its products, aerated drinks, candy, artificial syrups, sugar, and Junk food: Burger, pizza, samosa, vada etc., pastries and desserts. Bakery items: Biscuits, breads, cookies, puffs etc.

Adding good carbs to your diet and lowering your carb intake can help you maintain your blood glucose levels better.

The following foods **have no or negligible carbs 0-5 g** and they have very little impact on blood glucose levels.

- All vegetables
- Green leafy vegetables
- Nuts (most of them)
- Spices
- Eggs
- Seafood
- Meat and poultry
- Fats (Oil, butter and ghee)
- Cheese

Though low in carbohydrates, butter, oil, ghee, red meat are high in fat and hence need to be taken in restricted amounts.

There is a BIG difference between the natural, wholesome, 'good' carbs our bodies are designed to eat and the unnatural, highly processed, refined 'bad' carbs which many of us consume on a daily basis! Understanding the differences between 'good' carbs and 'bad' carbs can make all the difference.

Let's take a look at refined carbs or bad carbs

Bad carbs are refined, processed foods that have all or most of their **natural nutrients and fibre removed** in order to make them taste better and become more "consumer-friendly". The more refined the food, the worse it is for you.

> Refined Flour (maida) and table sugar are not the healthiest options as they spike your blood glucose levels quickly and also increase your blood triglyceride levels.

Listed below are the Bad Carbs

- Polished rice
- Maida or refined flour and its products
- Aerated drinks or soft drinks
- Candy
- Artificial syrups
- Sugar
- Pastries and desserts like gulab jamun, jalebi etc.
- Bakery items – biscuits, bread, pav, cookies, puffs

Processed/Refined carb foods provide large amounts of 'empty' calories (calories with little or no nutritional value). If you eat these foods in excess on a regular basis, your body will quickly turn them into body fat leading to obesity which in turn decreases your insulin effectiveness (causing insulin resistance).

Because of this, most of the processed carbs you eat wreak havoc on your natural hormone levels. Insulin production, goes haywire as the body attempts to process the huge amounts of starches and simple sugars contained in a typical 'bad carb'-based meal. This leads to dramatic fluctuations in blood glucose levels – a big reason why you often feel lethargic after eating high-carb meals. Since it is low in protein and fibre, it offers low satiety value, making you hungry soon after your meal.

> *It is becoming increasingly evident that the abundance of processed carbs and unhealthy trans-fats found in so many foods is a major cause of many of our modern chronic health problems!*

Real life example

Shruti (name changed) has Type 2 diabetes and is on oral anti-diabetes medications. She complained of regular bouts of low and high blood glucose levels. When she came to me for a consultation, I realized that her eating pattern had changed after she joined work. She socialised more often with her colleagues and business associates. Whenever she ate pizzas for dinner, her blood glucose levels were fine after 2 hours that is during bedtime but would run high late into the night. This is because fats take longer to digest and the blood glucose spikes up after 3–4 hours.

I counselled her about eating right during such times. She could choose a thin crust whole wheat pizza with lots of vegetable toppings and go slow on the cheese. This would not spike her blood glucose levels and also she could cut out the extra calories.

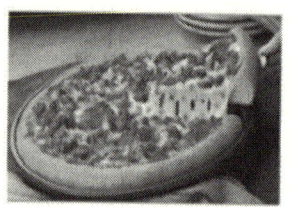 VS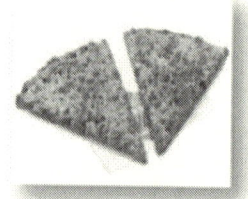

12 Inch Medium Pan Pizza

1 slice (cheese) = 240 calories and 27g carbs

12 Inch Thin "N" Crispy Pizza

1 slice = 190 calories and 22g carbs

Choose thin crust over thick crust, vegetable toppings over meat toppings, and hold the extra cheese

If she is eating popcorn at a movie, she could choose classic popcorn over flavoured, cheese or caramel popcorn. She followed this advice diligently and managed her blood glucose levels well even while eating out.

Regular consumption of large amounts of simple sugar, low-fibre, nutritionally-poor 'bad carbs' eventually leads to a much higher risk of obesity, cancer, heart disease, and other long-term complications.

While you can enjoy these unhealthy foods occasionally, you should not make them a regular feature in your meal plan. Also the term 'occasionally' does not mean you enjoy pizzas once a month and simultaneously also feast on food items such as samosas, vadas, ice cream or nankhatais with tea occasionally in the same month.

Occasional indulgence would also mean being true to yourself and only occasionally indulging in the food that you crave the most in a suitable portion size.

Real life example

I met Kedar (name changed), a 32-year-old working professional who has diabetes and is obese. He came to me for a consultation to lose weight and manage his diabetes.

When I asked him about his eating schedule, Kedar said, "Ma'am, I am a foodie and can live on a chicken roll, shawarma, vada pav or a samosa pav for lunch. That's the easiest to get and simplest to binge on. Also it keeps me full for a longer duration of time." And when I asked him about his dinner habits, he proudly said, "I eat a complete meal at dinner which consists of dal rice, chapatti, and vegetable cooked at home."

The dinner was fine, his eating habits during the day needed some changes. Throughout the consultation he displayed displeasure over the options that I gave him. He had a lot of excuses, he did not want to carry a big dabba and travel to the office. He had to leave early so the food was not ready when he left and so on and so forth. Finally, he settled on eating home-cooked lunch which could be prepared late and be sent to his office through a dabba wala. I suggested healthy options to choose from when he ate out and allowed him an occasional indulgence to avoid food cravings.

When I met him after a week there was no change in his weight or his blood glucose levels. I went through his meal log which he had maintained in his diary, he did have home-cooked food for all the three meals.

Additionally, he had a samosa and a vada pav on Monday evening, a piece of cake and a croissant on his friend's birthday on Wednesday, and on Saturday he had a marathon meeting in the office and had no choice but to binge on a slice of pizza, garlic bread and French fries.

He very gently told me, "I had **only occasionally indulged.**" By his understanding, he had a vada pav only once this week (compared to eating two vada pavs every day), it was just a piece of cake and a croissant, only a single slice of pizza, garlic bread and medium fries which he could not avoid in the board meeting. He did try his best to control the portion sizes but the indulgence was definitely not occasional hence his blood glucose levels were not under control this week.

I asked him to stay away from outside food only for a week and monitor his blood glucose levels more frequently. I also asked him to exercise and have his medications on time. He was willing to give it a try this time.

He came back to me with a smile on his face as his blood glucose levels showed a significant change and he was feeling lighter and happier.

People have their own definition of 'occasional'. But when you try to redefine your occasional indulgence or portion size, remember you are cheating only yourself and you are only harming your own body. It may not show immediately but it will creep up in the long run.

I do allow my patients to cheat but that means eating any one bad carb only once a week at one meal and that too when they are active. I also ask them to include fibre along with it like vegetables, salad, sautéed vegetable or stir fry.

Let's take a look at the 'good' carbs

Complex carbohydrates are good carbs because they offer many potential benefits to the human body.

They are high in fibre offering a higher satiety value thus aiding in weight loss by keeping you full for a longer period of time. They generally have a lower glycemic load, which means that you will get lower amounts of glucose released at a more consistent rate (maintain blood glucose stability) and keep you going throughout the day. They are rich in the essential vitamins and minerals which the body requires to maintain good health and prevent diseases.

The following food types are generally considered to be good carbs and should make up most of your entire carb intake:

- Vegetables
- Whole fruits
- Whole pulses and sprouts
- Whole grain cereals

Picking complex carbohydrates over simple carbohydrates is a matter of making some simple substitutions when it comes to your meals. Choose unpolished rice instead of polished rice, durum wheat or quinoa pasta instead of plain white pasta, fruits over fruit juice, daliya or broken wheat over maida.

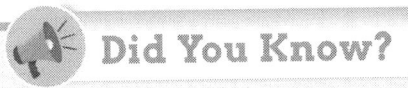

Buckwheat (kuttu) is not a cereal but a pseudo grain. It is commonly consumed during fasting as a porridge, upma, dhokla or dosa in some parts of India and can be consumed by people having diabetes.

> Include the good carbs in your diet for a healthier, fitter, alert and energetic "YOU".

Some Do's and Don'ts

1. Try to cut out as much 'unhealthy food' from your diet as possible. This includes all salted chips, bakery foods, candy, soft drinks, fried foods etc.

2. Avoid or limit your intake of refined flour, baked goods, including white bread, naan, doughnuts, khari, puffs, nankhatais, biscuits, brownies, cakes, etc. Also, avoid consuming processed, high-sugar (high-fructose corn syrup) breakfast cereals – stick to whole grain cereals and oatmeal instead.

3. Buy a variety of fresh fruits and include at least one or two servings in a day.

4. Snack on a fruit or cut-up vegetables when hungry– a single apple can easily curb hunger.

5. Eat a serving of green vegetables at least twice a day. Include salads and unstrained soups in your diet. Also, eat a variety of other colourful vegetables as often as possible to get your dose of antioxidants.

6. Use nuts and seeds as healthy, portable snacks you can carry anywhere.

7. Eat a serving of sprouts made from whole pulses like green gram, moth beans, brown chana, at least once or twice a day. Sprouts are considered to be one of the most nutritionally 'powerful' protein-rich foods available.

8. Always choose the whole grain option when it comes to bread, cereals, biscuits, pasta, etc. Just make sure that 'whole grain' is the first word in the ingredients list.

To know if a packaged food is made of simple or complex carbohydrates look at the label and if the first ingredient is whole grain flour, eg: whole wheat flour, it is likely to be a complex carbohydrate.

Real life example

My patient, Krutika (name changed), is a foodie and likes to try various cuisines. She has diabetes. She came to me and said, "I will do everything you tell me but don't tell me not to eat this, not to eat that. I love pasta and cannot live without it but every time I eat Alfredo Pasta, my blood glucose levels rise rapidly." She was stressed as she had to give up her favourite food which was further troubling her blood glucose levels.

I tried to explain to her that pasta was made from refined flour and the sauce that she prepared using cream and refined flour were bad carbs, hence her blood glucose levels would increase after a few hours of eating. I suggested, "You can eat the Alfredo Pasta, but you need to follow some instructions. Before having the pasta, you need to first have a bowl of vegetable soup or salad." Krutika said, "Kuch bhi (anything) for eating my pasta."

I then gave her instructions on which pasta to choose and how to cook it if she is making it at home. I asked her to use durum wheat or quinoa pasta and cook the Alfredo sauce using 1 tsp olive oil, 1 tbsp wheat flour and 1 cup low-fat milk along with all the condiments. Along with the pasta, I asked her to add a lot of colourful vegetables like broccoli, red, yellow and green bell peppers, baby corn, mushrooms, and baby spinach. She said, she'd give it a try.

She came to me the next time, happy and contented. She said that the advice had helped. She felt very satiated and satisfied after eating the pasta.

Replacing bad carbs with good carbs made a huge difference to her blood glucose levels.

> Choosing carbs wisely is important to remain healthy and maintain normal blood sugar levels.

People generally believe or are told to eat small frequent meals to lose weight and in the bargain keep eating meals rich in carb every two to three hours. This spikes up insulin levels and increases fat accumulation. Increased body fat further increases insulin resistance, thus causing blood glucose levels to rise.

It is thus advisable to choose low carb options like vegetable sticks, curd/plain yogurt, cheese (not more than one cube/one slice), cottage cheese/paneer (less than 50 g), egg, nuts, cheese, tofu, soy nuts, clear soups (watch the sauces), salad with paneer/egg/chicken (watch the dressings), salted lassi/buttermilk, sprouts, makhana (in prescribed amounts) as between-meal options which will not spike up blood glucose levels.

Disclaimer: *This advice is for people with no medical conditions and not for people with diabetes on insulin or oral anti-diabetes drugs which cause low blood glucose levels/hypoglycaemia. Please consult a qualified dietitian for a customised meal plan.*

Should fats or carbs be avoided?

This question is asked quite often. Unlike olden times when for scientific, health or wellness related information, one used to refer to books, research articles and seek advice from health care professionals, the source of information now is the internet and social media. People have become more confused than ever, because of the conflicting information available on such sources which may or may not be backed by research. Also because of evolving science over time and areas of uncertainty in the scientific literature, the concept of nutrients is at times very confusing for everyone. Fat and carbohydrates are the most confusing nutrients.

World Health Organisation (WHO) recommends a total fat intake of 20–35% of the diet. Nuts and seeds must be incorporated in the diet as they are sources of healthy fats and provide protection to the heart. Fats are also an essential part of the diet as they help in absorption of essential fat-soluble vitamins namely Vitamins A, D, E and K.

People get carried away by the latest trends. Low carbohydrate diets have been the focus of considerable interest since the last few years. Low carbohydrate diets are high in fats and therefore they can be termed as Low Carb High Fat diets [LCHF, Keto Diet (20–50 g carbs per day)].

The Keto diet was initially used as a therapeutic diet for patients with epilepsy but recent studies indicate the short-term improvements in glycemic control, weight loss, and heart disease risk by following a Low Carb High Fat diet.

If you wish to embark on a low carb or a ketogenic diet, kindly inform your doctor and dietitian. They will do a thorough assessment of your health and let you know if you can follow such a diet for a short period or you shouldn't. They will also review your medications, blood reports and customise a meal plan and prescription to prevent low blood glucose episodes and any other complications.

Facts to note

- Any diet type resulting in reduced energy intake will result in weight loss and related favourable metabolic and functional changes

- Short-term Low Carb High Fat (LCHF) diets studies show both favourable and less desirable effects
- Increases the number of hypoglycemic (low blood glucose) episodes
- Increases bad blood cholesterol (LDL cholesterol) levels and therefore risk for heart disease in the long run (Leow et al, Diabetic medicine, 2018)
- Sustained adherence to a ketogenic LCHF diet appears to be difficult
- There is a lack of data supporting long-term efficacy, safety and health benefits of LCHF diets

The negative aspects of low carbohydrate diets include nutritional deficiencies, namely those commonly found in unprocessed carbohydrate foods including vitamins, minerals, dietary fibre, and phytochemical with antioxidant properties. In conclusion, what is more important than the quantity of carbohydrates is the type of carbohydrates. There is now accumulating evidence that unprocessed carbohydrates, including whole grains, fruit, vegetables, and legumes, have health benefits and those from refined sources, including white bread and white rice and particularly sugar and sugar-sweetened beverages (aerated drinks), are associated with increased risk of obesity, heart disease and type 2 diabetes.

A study published in a well-known journal found that diets both low (< 40% energy) and high (> 70% energy) in carbohydrates were linked with an increase in mortality (death) while moderate consumers of carbohydrates (50–55% of energy) had the lowest risk of mortality. **Hence eating carbohydrates in moderation seems to be optimal for health and longevity.**

Children and adolescents are not recommended to follow the ketogenic diet as it impacts growth and development. Studies have shown that it causes stunting of growth and impacts developmental milestones adversely.

We have our patients reverse diabetes and improve blood glucose levels even on a moderate carbohydrate (50%) meal plan.

Another commonly asked question is should I go gluten-free?

The humble wheat has become a villain today and many people are going off wheat completely because of gluten in the pursuit to lose weight and achieve better blood glucose control. Gluten is a protein present in wheat and wheat products, barley, rye and spelt. In people with celiac disease, there is an immune reaction to gluten causing diarrhoea, abdominal pain, bloating etc., hence wheat and other gluten-containing foods are avoided.

Many people believe that oats has gluten, but this isn't true. Oats do not have gluten but could have been processed in a factory which has processed wheat and its products.. Hence for people with celiac disease, it is recommended that they buy oats which is labelled gluten-free.

People think they lose weight and blood glucose improves after giving up gluten, but the truth is that they stop eating unhealthy foods which also happen to contain gluten like bread, biscuits, burgers, pizzas, naans, parathas, roomali roti, rusks (toast) and khari made from refined flour (made with maida). By doing this they lose weight and see an improvement in blood glucose levels. You do not need to go gluten-free unless advised by your doctor/dietitian. You can enjoy wheat, barley and its products guilt-free. But remember **"Moderation is key."**

> Follow a diet which is nutritionally balanced, sustainable, easy to follow and is light on your pockets.

 Did You Know?

As per a recent study published, restricting calories to less than 800–1000 calories in adults under strict medical supervision of a qualified dietitian and doctor has shown to reverse type 2 diabetes. A meal replacer (shakes/meals/bars) which is nutritionally adequate may be recommended in such situations. They help provide the body with the necessary nutrients while restricting calories. Speak to your doctor or consult a qualified dietitian for more information on "Reversal of Type 2 Diabetes"

Here is a real life journey shared by a patient who reversed Type 2 Diabetes – Anju Paul

MIRACLES do happen!! In my case, my diabetes was reversed.

I was detected with Type 2 diabetes with an HbA1c of 7.5 and was overweight in October 2015, I got scared and rushed to my dietitian who taught me the discipline of eating and staying fit.

I learnt from my diabetologist and dietitian that if I wish to get rid of diabetes, I had to reduce inches especially around my waist and visceral fat.

I was determined to lose all the extra flab that I had accumulated over the years. To stay focused towards achieving my goal even during the festive season or while going out with family and friends, I never hesitated to tell people that I am working on my diet and I choose to eat only healthy food. This helped me in two ways:

1. No one forced me to eat more.
2. My friends and relatives helped me to select healthier food options and there were times when they also chose to eat healthier food. (Good health for them too!)

My dietitian discussed my lifestyle and eating pattern and made very simple and easy to follow changes in my diet.

My daily food intake has not changed much except that I have switched to fibre rich foods. No more maida (refined flour) for me. I have cut down on my sugar and sweet intake. I indulge in fried foods occasionally. I now have salads with every meal. I consciously add protein to my meal. And above all I keep my body hydrated by drinking enough water during the day. I de-stress my body by giving it adequate rest by maintaining my sleep schedule. These minor changes have changed my life.

Regular exercise is now a part of my everyday schedule. I go for a walk daily and also do Zumba twice a week.

I can now proudly say that I used to have diabetes which is now reversed. My present HbA1c is 5.5 and I lost five inches on my waist, and achieved normal visceral fat levels. I am off all medicines too. I can just say that eating right can make immense changes to your body.

EAT HEALTHY, FEEL HEALTHY!!

CHAPTER 06
The Story of Numbers: Glycemic Index and Glycemic Load

The story of numbers

People these days are increasingly concerned about their health and show immense interest in understanding newer concepts. One such that I have observed is people are keen to know more about is 'Glycemic Index' and its importance in blood glucose control.

Glycemic index, also known as (GI), is basically the effect of food on your blood glucose levels. Carbohydrates from different foods lead to different blood glucose responses.

Some foods lead to an immediate spike in blood glucose levels while some foods get digested slowly to give a sustained release of glucose over time without causing a sudden spike in the blood glucose levels.

Glycemic index measures the amount of increase in circulating blood glucose caused by a carbohydrate-containing food. It ranks foods based on the blood glucose response they evoke. The reference meal is usually glucose or white bread.

The consumption of high glycemic index foods results in higher and more rapid increases in blood glucose levels than the consumption of low glycemic index foods. The consumption of low glycemic index foods results in lower but more sustained increase in blood glucose and will not trigger a dramatic spike in blood glucose levels.

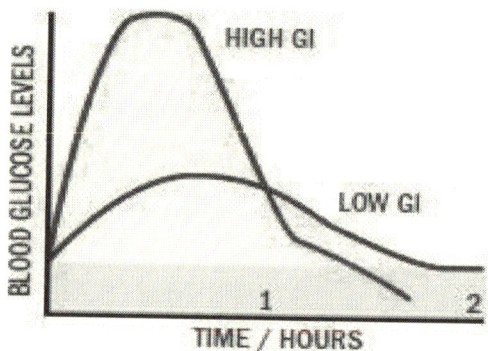

This is how the glycemic index of the food affects the blood glucose level in the body.

Glycemic index is categorized as:

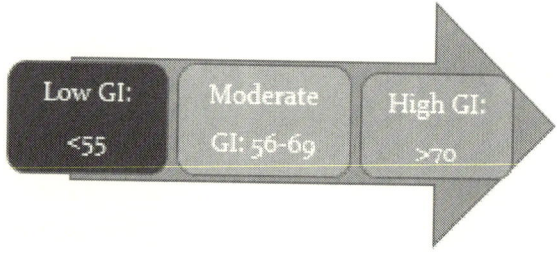

Glycemic Index of foods

Low GI (< 55)	Moderate GI (56–69)	High GI (> 70)
All bran	Whole wheat bread Whole wheat roti	White bread
Long grain basmati rice	Short grain basmati rice	
Pearl Barley	Beetroot	Corn and Cornflakes
		Mashed potato
Rajma, lentils, Bengal gram, black gram, green gram	Pineapple, papaya, mango (depends on the ripeness)	Baked potato
Soybean	Jowar	Dates

Apple, Pear, Orange	Bajra	Watermelon
Curd (plain)	Quinoa	Glucose
Ice cream (*high in fat)		Ragi (nachni)
Chicken, fish		Short Grain White Rice (ambemohar)
Parboiled rice		Medium Grain White Rice (Sona masuri, Surti kolum)
Steel-Cut Oats and Rolled Oats		Quick Instant Oats Noodles

Reference: Nazni. P and Ravinder Singh, Meta analysis study of glycemic index of various food groups, e-ISSN 2320 –7876 www.ijfans.com, Vol.3, Iss.4, Jul-Sep 2014

Real life example

My patient Ramadevi (name changed) had diabetes, and loved to have upma (semolina) for breakfast. She noticed that every time she ate upma for breakfast, her post-breakfast blood glucose levels were high.

She came to me for consultation and said, "Ma'am, whenever I eat upma my blood glucose levels increase immediately. I make upma for my family but I avoid eating with the fear that my blood glucose levels would rise."

I explained to Ramadevi that upma was made from rawa or semolina and has a high glycemic index so the glucose levels rise immediately. I asked her to add vegetables and soya granules/sprouts/roasted peanut or groundnut powder to the upma. This would increase the fibre and protein content and lower the glycemic index. She can also substitute rawa with daliya or broken wheat as it is coarser and therefore has a lower glycemic index than rawa.

She could also have a handful of unsalted almonds or a whole boiled egg before the upma. This would help maintain the post-meal blood glucose levels in the target range.

Ramadevi followed the advice and her blood glucose levels were much better.

Factors Affecting Glycemic Index

There is no need to get scared with the numbers or the glycemic index and stop eating foods that have a high glycemic index. You need to understand the factors that affect the glycemic index and ways of reducing the glycemic index of the food. Yes, you heard me right.

1) Cooking time

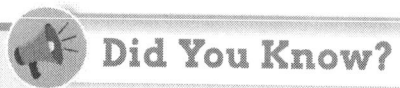 **Did You Know?**

A recent study showed that rice chewed fifteen times produced a significantly lower post meal glucose spike than when chewed thirty times.

Longer cooking times may increase the glucose increasing capacity of the food by breaking down the starch or carbohydrate and allowing it to pass through the body more quickly when consumed.

Overcooked rice will have a higher glycemic index compared to rice cooked till slightly grainy and tender for a shorter time. Cook rice and drain off the water to remove the excess starch.

Pasta cooked for 5–10 minutes has a slightly lower GI than pasta cooked longer.

Starchy foods should not be overcooked.

Real life example

I met a south Indian lady, Laxmi (name changed), who was a 37-year-old homemaker. She was diagnosed with diabetes and her blood glucose levels were all over the place. In spite of all the medications given by the doctor, her blood glucose levels would never be in the normal range. She approached me to help plan her diet.

When I spoke to her she said, "My staple diet is rice, so I eat rice for both the meals." When I asked her, "How much rice do you eat?" She said, "Very little," showing a cup size quantity of rice with her palms. Later, after a while of talking to her and understanding her routine, I found out that her quantity of little was as much as a dinner plate.

I counselled her on the importance of controlling portions and asked her to use unpolished rice, parboiled rice or brown rice, and educated her on the method of preparing it. I also advised her to include fibre and protein-rich foods with rice to blunt the blood glucose response. She went back very happy that she could eat rice. In a few days, she reported that her blood glucose levels were in control in spite of eating rice.

2) Cooking methods

Steaming or moist heat cooking at a temperature of about 50°C in the presence of water causes an increase in glycemic index due to gelatinization of starch.

For instance, raw carrots have a low glycemic index while cooked carrots and beetroot have a much higher glycemic index compared to raw ones.

Only in case of sweet potatoes, studies have shown that boiling decreased the glycemic index when compared to frying, baking, and roasting.

3) Acidity

The more acidic a food is, the lower is the glycemic index. For e.g. pickled food or foods containing vinegar or lemon juice have a lower glycemic index.

Squeezing lemon or adding vinegar to food helps lower the glycemic index.

Sourdough bread easily available at big supermarkets today use lactobacillus or lactic acid culture as part of the leavening process and have a lower glycemic index than white bread.

4) Overall food composition

It is possible to modulate the rapid increase in blood glucose brought about by food that has a high glycemic index by consuming it with a food that has a low glycemic index.

Foods high in protein, fat and fibre normally have a low glycemic index. So combining them with high glycemic index foods can lead to a slower increase in blood glucose levels.

For example, having paneer (cottage cheese)/cheese and vegetables with a slice of bread would decrease the glycemic index of the meal containing bread.

Combining rice with pulses/legumes helps lower the glycemic index of the meal.

> Balance-out the effects of a high GI food by eating it with low GI foods such as those high in protein and fiber like pulses, beans, curd, buttermilk, cottage cheese, lean meat, whole grain cereals, vegetables and high fiber fruits.

Ref: Mahan, L. Kathleen., Escott-Stump, Sylvia., Raymond, Janice L. Krause, Marie V. (12th Eds.) (2012) Krause's food and the nutrition care process/St. Louis, Mo.: Elsevier/Saunders; pg 766–799

To understand better, poha or rice flakes is a popular Indian breakfast item. Hand-pounded poha has a high fibre content and moderate glycemic index, however the poha available today is machine-made and has a high glycemic index which causes your blood glucose levels to spike rapidly. This does not mean you stop eating poha, you can add a lot of vegetables like capsicum, cabbage and peanuts to slow down the increase in blood sugar levels. Follow the traditional practice of squeezing lemon on the poha to lower the glycemic index.

Curd/Buttermilk or Egg can be had along with the poha. Have the buttermilk or the egg first and then have the poha to blunt the spike in blood glucose levels.

A Maharashtrian recipe called dadpe pohe is also a good breakfast option for people with diabetes.

Here is the recipe of dadpe pohe

Serves: 4

Ingredients

Hand-pounded poha	6 handfuls
Onions, finely chopped	½ cup
Tomatoes, finely chopped	½ cup
Capsicum, finely chopped	¼ cup
Lemon juice	3 tsp
Coriander, finely chopped	¼ cup
Green chillies	2 no.
Salt	To taste
Fresh grated Coconut	1 tbsp
Peanuts/Groundnuts, coarsely ground	2 tbsp

Method:

- Put the hand-pounded poha in a large plate. Add onions, tomatoes, capsicum, salt, coconut, peanuts and green chillies in poha.

- Mix everything with your hand. Pohe will become wet due to the vegetables and salt. For flavour you can give a tadka of mustard, asafoetida (hing) and curry leaves.
- Squeeze lemon to further reduce the glycemic index.
- Garnish it with coriander leaves and serve.

Ragi/Finger millet/Nachni/Nagli is often a millet of choice for people with diabetes. Most of the patients we know, on the advice of self-proclaimed diet experts, shun wheat phulkas for a ragi roti/bhakri, they swap dalia porridge with ragi malt porridge or finish off an entire packet of ragi biscuits thinking it is healthy and will do no harm to their blood glucose levels.

Many do not know that Ragi has a high glycemic index of 84 and it shoots up blood glucose levels rapidly. Does that mean you give up eating ragi? The answer is NO!

Ragi has a myriad of health benefits and is often the first meal given to children. It is also the millet of choice for the geriatric population. One can make a ragi dosa by mixing ragi with urad dal, adding grated vegetables and buttermilk to make the batter. This becomes a complete meal as it has all the food groups. Adding udad dal, buttermilk and vegetables lower the glycemic index. The ragi powder available outside which we use to make porridge spikes up blood glucose rapidly. It is best to use ragi to make a dosa or an idli rather than in porridge form.

Over the years of interacting with many patients with diabetes, I have seen there are many people who feel sad about giving up their favourite foods as their blood glucose levels get affected. In most of the cases you can enjoy your favourite foods by making modifications in the ingredients or in the cooking method.

> Low to moderate glycemic index millets such as sanwa (barnyard millet), kangni (foxtail millet), bajra (pearl millet), kodon (kodu), sama (little millet) and jowar (sorghum) must be included in the diet.

5) Resistant Starch

Resistant starch resists digestion in the small intestine and acts like fibre in the large intestine. As it resists digestion, foods containing this type of starch have a low glycemic index.

Resistant starch is naturally found in unripe bananas, raw potatoes, seeds and pulses. Cooking these foods causes changes in the starch, removing the resistant starch and making it easily digestible.

Raw banana flour has a higher content of resistant starch and can be used in different recipes. It is gaining a lot of popularity in Indian cuisine and is easily available in most supermarkets or e-commerce websites

Resistant starch is formed when starch-containing foods are cooked and cooled, such as legumes, rice, potatoes, corn, pasta.

We are all used to eating food that is freshly cooked but some foods like rice, potato, sweet potato, pasta and pulses when cooked, cooled for 24 hours and reheated at low temperatures less than 50 degrees centigrade/130 degrees Fahrenheit helps to retain the resistant starch.

Cooling of cooked white rice increases resistant starch content.

Cooked white rice cooled for 24 hours at 4°C then reheated has a lower glycemic response compared with freshly cooked white rice. (Ref: Sonia S, et al. Asia Pac J Clin Nutr. 2015). This resistant starch has a lower glycemic index and thus helps to reduce sudden spikes in post-meal blood glucose levels.

Remember to reheat at low temperatures as heating the food at higher temperatures will again convert the starch into a form that is digestible to us, thereby increasing the glycemic index.

Real life example

Vidya (name changed) had diabetes and loved to eat the humble south Indian food sambar rice and potato vegetable. Rice and potato both have a high glycemic index hence would immediately raise her blood glucose levels.

When she came to me for a consultation, she said, "I know you may laugh at me for asking this silly question but I just love my staple diet of sambar rice and absolutely miss eating potato. I also know that having diabetes, it is not very good for my health. I tried swapping it with brown rice and cooking raw banana instead of potatoes but frankly, I did not enjoy it."

I gave her a meal plan with all the healthy food items that she liked. When she was going through her meal plan she saw one bowl of sambar rice on one weekday and potato on another day in her meal plan.

Vidya said with a very heavy heart, "Ma'am its ok. I just shared with you that I miss eating these foods but I am ok with not eating them." I told her, "You can eat this food provided you follow two things." She looked at me in surprise as if I was going to ask for something too much. I said, "You need to maintain your portions that means you can eat one cup of rice with sambar which has a lot of vegetables added to it. Secondly, you can cook the rice a day prior, refrigerate for 24 hours and reheat at low temperature the next day before eating."

"The same goes with potatoes; you can boil your potatoes a day in advance, refrigerate for 24 hours and cook it on the next day. Along with that you need to monitor your blood glucose levels regularly." Surprised, Vidya asked me if I was talking about 'Basi chawal' which is leftover rice. When I explained to her about how resistant starch is developed and how it would help reduce the glycemic index of the starchy food, she was more than happy to eat that 'Basi Chawal'.

Her blood sugar monitoring log and diet log showed how her blood glucose was under control while she relished her favourite food.

 Did You Know?

Cook starchy foods, cool at 4 degrees C for 24 hours and reheat at low temperatures (less than 130 degrees F or 50°C) to increase the amount of resistant starch and thus lower the Glycemic index.

Drying, dehydration, germination, popping, puffing, flaking and fermentation processes decrease the resistant starch and increase the glycemic index. Hence, we observe that rice flakes, popcorn and idli, dosa tend to increase the blood glucose levels.

6) Particle size and variety of grain

When starchy foods are ground, their particles become much finer, making their digestion easier and increasing the glycemic index. This is what happens to cereals when they are ground into flour.

Rice flour, accordingly, has a higher glycemic index than rice itself. Similarly, more the processing, lower the fibre content, finer the particles, higher is the glycemic index.

For instance, wheat has a low glycemic index while maida (white flour) has a high glycemic index.

Wheat < broken wheat < semolina < wheat flour < maida

Even the variety of grain affects glycemic index. Long grain white rice has a lower glycemic index compared to short grain white rice. Short grain rice such as Ambemohar, Sona masuri, Surti kolum have a high glycemic index while long grain basmati has a medium glycemic index and brown rice has a low glycemic index. Aged rice (purana chawal or raw rice stored for a long time) has a lower glycemic index and hence we have seen our grandparents and mothers buying old or aged rice.

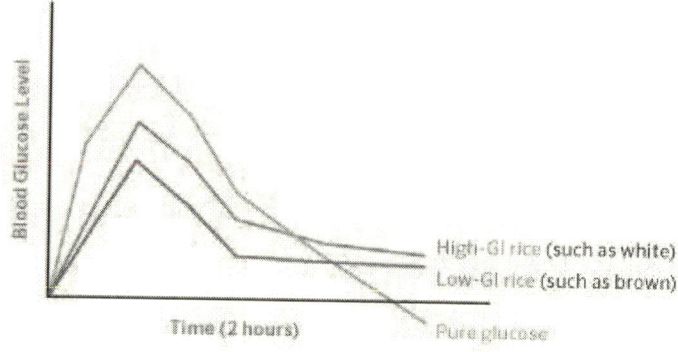

Reference: *International Journal of Food Sciences and Nutrition 63(2):178–83 • September 2011*

Ref: *Shobana Shanmugam et al*

Many whole grains and pulses have a lower glycemic index as the fibrous coat around beans, seeds, and plant cell walls in whole grains acts as a physical barrier, slowing access of digestive enzymes to break down the carbohydrate.

7) Physical form

The more processed a food, the higher is its glycemic index. For example, instant oatmeal has a higher glycemic index of 79, whereas steel-cut or rolled oats has a lower glycemic index of 55. Therefore when buying oats, always read the label and look for rolled or steel-cut oats. Do not buy instant oats as it will spike up the blood glucose levels rapidly.

> Always add whole grains, legumes and unprocessed foods like broken wheat, steel cut oats, rolled oats, barley, bajra, jowar, and pulses in your diet.

Fruits

The riper the fruit, higher will be its glycemic Index. Patients with diabetes should not store fruits for a long time and avoid consuming overripe fruits.

For instance, green firm un-ripened banana has a low glycemic index while a ripened banana, yellow with brown spots has a higher glycemic index.

Fruit juice has a higher glycemic index than the whole fruit and hence must be avoided.

8) Food Order

How you consume your meal also affects the glycemic response. Several studies have shown that if you eat protein and fibre first followed by carbs or starch, the glycemic response will be slower. For example if you have chicken, fish, paneer or dal with vegetables first followed by rice or chapatti, the post-meal blood glucose level spike will be blunted.

Having a handful of nuts before you start your meal has shown to blunt the post meal blood glucose spikes.

You need to make wise choices while selecting food options. The truth is that if you eat a nutritious and balanced diet that consists of whole grains, vegetables, lean proteins, and dairy, you will be eating a lower glycemic index diet.

Also adding proteins and fibre to every meal can help you bring down the glycemic index and improve your blood glucose levels. In case you have a kidney issue or any co-morbid conditions you need to consult your dietitian or doctor before making changes to your meal plan.

Glycemic Load

Glycemic index indicates how rapidly a particular carbohydrate from food causes a rise in blood glucose levels. It does not give any information on how much of that carbohydrate is present in a serving of that food.

Glycemic load gives you the actual picture of the effect of carbohydrate from food and is a more accurate indicator of the meals overall effect on blood glucose levels.

For example: The glycemic index of 1 cup (150 g) watermelon is 72. This makes it a high glycemic index food. Although watermelon has a high glycemic index, but compared to other fruits, it doesn't have as much carbohydrate because it is mainly water. The small amount of carbohydrate in watermelon is absorbed very quickly making it a high glycemic index food, but because the carb content is very low, it will not have much effect on the blood glucose levels, so in terms of impact, it is very low. This is termed as 'Glycemic Load'.

The glycemic load, also known as (GL) of a food is calculated by multiplying the glycemic index by the amount of carbohydrate in grams provided by a food and dividing the total by 100.

Glycemic Load is categorized as:

Low GL < 10

Moderate GL: 11–19

High GL: > 20

So calculating the GL of watermelon:

Glycemic Load= Glycemic index X carbohydrate (g) in food portion consumed GI: 72 and carb content in ½ cup watermelon – 6 gm

Glycemic Load: [72 x 6]/100 = 4

Glycemic load of 1 cup of watermelon is 4 which falls in the low GL category and so it will not have much effect on blood glucose levels and can be taken safely in controlled portions.

Apple

GI – 40 and carb content in 1 apple – 15 g

Glycemic Load: [40 x 15]/100 = 6 (low Glycemic load)

When considering a low or high glycemic index food, you need to consider how much carbohydrate a portion of food contains and thus considering glycemic load of food along with glycemic index gives a better idea of glycemic response.

 Frequently Asked Question

Can a person with diabetes consume coconut water?

Coconut water is a natural electrolyte and is the richest source of potassium, hence recommended for people with high blood pressure. However people are often confused about its recommendation in diabetes.

Nutritional content of Coconut water (200 ml):

Calories: 30 cals

Protein: 0.52 g

Carbohydrate: 6 g

Fat: 0.32 g

Glycemic Index – 67±18.9 (moderate)

Glycemic Load – 7±2.0 (low)

Though the carbohydrate content is low, glycemic index is moderate and glycemic load is low, it does not have fiber-like other fruits. Therefore people with diabetes can occasionally consume coconut water instead of a fruit preferably with the malai (coconut meat) or a fistful of nuts to prevent the spike in blood glucose levels. It is best if consumed before or during a workout.

Real life journey shared by Mehak, mother of Meera who is a 20-month-old Type 1 diabetes

My daughter Meera is 20 months old and has been diagnosed with type 1 diabetes since the past few months. Being a little child it was very difficult for me to plan her meals and manage her hypoglycaemia and hyperglycaemia.

She is on 5 shots a day (3 short-acting insulin injection i.e. before meals and 2 long-acting insulin injection i.e. in the morning and at bedtime) and would have blood glucose fluctuations which were becoming difficult to manage. She had low blood glucose levels and when treated would later become very high.

When I met my dietitian, she helped me plan her meal schedule.

She educated me on the method of cooking potato and rice to increase the resistant starch and thanks to that my daughter can now enjoy her potato and rice without her blood glucose spiking up.

She offered options of mid-meals snacks such as makhana/jowar puff/ragi puffs instead of her high-carb options like bread and biscuits. Similarly in the evening she swapped her carb meals with paneer and vegetables or tikki.

Just by making small changes in her mid-meal snacks helped me manage my daughter's blood glucose levels in a better way. Understanding the meal requirement and insulin dosage is very individualistic and my dietitian has helped us manage and balance the two.

Hypothyroidism and Its Dietary Management

CHAPTER 07

Hypothyroidism is a disorder that occurs when the thyroid gland does not produce enough thyroid hormones. Once diagnosed by your doctor by clinical examination and series of blood tests, thyroid hormone medications may be started to supplement low thyroid levels. It is also called synthetic thyroid hormone.

Here are a few guidelines to follow to ensure that your thyroid gland works to its optimum levels

- Always use iodized salt.
- You may have heard people asking you to avoid certain foods. Yes, goitrogen containing foods such as cabbage, cauliflower, broccoli, flax seeds, walnuts, soy & soy products combine with iodine and make it unavailable for the synthesis of the thyroid hormone. However, cooking neutralizes the goitrogens present in these foods, hence these foods in the cooked form can be consumed in recommended amounts.
- Hydrate yourself well with 8–10 glasses of water unless advised against by your doctor. It prevents constipation, fatigue and sugar cravings which are common complaints in hypothyroidism.

- Take your thyroid medication at the same time every day at least 40 minutes before eating food.

- Avoid taking your thyroid medication at the same time as walnuts, soybean flour, fibre, calcium or iron supplements or multivitamins containing iron, calcium supplements, antacids that contain aluminum, magnesium or calcium, some cholesterol-lowering drugs, such as those containing cholestyramine (Prevalite) and colestipol (Colestid). These foods and supplements may interfere with the absorption of the thyroid medication. It is recommended to keep a gap of four hours between the thyroid medication and these foods.

- Regular moderate intensity exercise will help to improve the thyroid function, promote sound sleep & increase stamina. An easy way to start exercising is to walk for 30 minutes a day. One can also try swimming, biking, or any other moderate-intensity activity. However, consult a doctor before embarking on any exercise regime

Foods to include
Protein sources like egg, fish, chicken, curd, and pulses
Whole-grains, legumes & pulses, fruits and vegetables
Selenium rich foods such as green gram, dry peas, brazil nuts, whole egg and amaranth leaves

Frequently Asked Question

Pink Salt, Black Salt, Sendha Namak – which one to use?

I have many patients asking me if pink, black, kala namak, sendha namak is better than white salt or regular table salt. Let me tell you that the amount of sodium in all the salts is almost the same. The mineral content in the other salts is miniscule (just 2%) to make any difference to our health. We can easily get them from the balanced diet that we eat.

CHAPTER 08: Hyperuricemia (High Uric Acid Levels)

We often see patients with obesity, prediabetes and diabetes having high uric acid levels.

Hyperuricemia occurs when there is an excessive amount of uric acid in the blood. High uric acid levels in severe cases can lead to a painful type of arthritis called gout.

Gout is a type of arthritis that causes swelling and pain in joints due to excessive accumulation of uric acid in blood.

Reasons for high uric acid levels are

- Dehydration
- Increased alcohol intake
- Purine rich foods
- Obesity/Metabolic Syndrome
- High fructose intake especially high-fructose corn syrup (HFCS) from packaged foods

Dietary guidelines:

- Being overweight is one of the major factors in increasing the risk for high uric acid levels. Thus, it is advisable to lose weight gradually.

- Include nutritionally balanced meals at regular intervals throughout the day.

- Include vitamin C rich food sources like gooseberry (amla), guava and oranges as it can help to lower uric acid levels.

- Dehydration is one of the causes of high uric acid levels. Stay well-hydrated. It is recommended to increase water consumption unless advised against doing so by your doctor.

- Restrict the consumption of fructose containing foods and beverages. Avoid foods that are sweetened with HFCS - high fructose corn syrup such as aerated drinks, juices, cereals, candy, pastries, donuts, cake and cookies. It is recommended to read food labels to understand if there is high fructose corn syrup as an ingredient in the packaged foods.

- Liver breaks down purines from food and produces a waste product called uric acid. Therefore, purine rich foods must be avoided.

- Stay physically active and exercise regularly. It is advisable to consult your doctor and dietitian before embarking on any exercise regime.

Foods to include and exclude

Food group	Foods to include	Foods to exclude
Cereal, millets and their products	Whole grain cereals & millets like sorghum (jowar), pearl millet (bajra), finger millet (ragi/ nachni), foxtail millet etc.	Yeast or yeast containing food products like bread and naan
Pulses and Legumes	Dals, Lentils, soy and soy products (in moderate amounts)	

Milk and Meat products	Low fat dairy products such as milk, curd, plain yogurt, cottage cheese (paneer), egg	Organ meats (heart, kidneys, liver, tongue), red meat, shrimps, mackerel, sardines, fish egg, sausages
Vegetables and Fruits	Seasonal fruits especially cherries	Purine rich foods like Peas, spinach, cauliflower, asparagus, brinjal, mushrooms, sapota (chickoo), custard apple (sitaphal)
Miscellaneous	Unsalted nuts and seeds	Aerated drinks, alcohol especially beer, sugar sweetened beverages, sugary foods, foods containing high fructose corn syrup.

In Summary

- *A well- balanced, alkaline diet which is low in purine rich foods, low in high fructose corn syrup with a focus on adequate hydration and reduction in alcohol intake is recommended in Hyperuricemia.*
- *Patients are encouraged to lose weight if overweight.*

CHAPTER 09 All about Carbohydrate, Protein and Fat Counting

This chapter is useful for patients on multiple daily insulin regime (basal bolus insulin therapy) or those on insulin pump therapy

Foods contain nutrients that are required by your body for good health. The nutrients that contribute to calories are carbohydrate, protein, and fat. Carbohydrates by far have the greatest short-term impact on your blood glucose levels more than protein or fat. Protein and fat take several hours (up to three to four hours) to show up as blood glucose, so they play a minor role in short-term blood glucose control. More on the impact of protein and fat later in this chapter.

Before we learn about carbohydrate counting, let us first understand the different types of insulins available today.

Basal insulin:

Intermediate/Long-acting insulin which keeps your blood glucose levels in range between meals, overnight and at fasting.

Examples: Lantus, Levemir, Tresiba, Toujeo, Insulatard (NPH), Huminsulin N

Bolus Insulin:

Short-acting, rapid-acting or fast-acting insulin is given to control post-meal blood glucose levels. This is called Food Bolus. It is also used to 'correct' an out of range blood glucose-correction bolus.

Examples: Actrapid, Huminsulin R, Apidra, Novorapid, Humalog, Fiasp

For people with Type 1 diabetes (on separate shots of bolus insulin – short-acting/rapid-acting with basal insulin – intermediate/long-acting insulin), carbohydrate counting is absolutely the key to maintaining tight control over your blood glucose levels. You count the carbohydrates in a meal you are about to eat and then adjust the amount of short-acting or rapid-acting insulin you inject or the "bolus" on your insulin pump to 'balance out' those carbohydrates as precisely as you can. By doing this, you are trying to mimic the healthy pancreas and release just the right amount of insulin to cover the carbohydrates you eat. With the right balance of carbohydrates and insulin, your blood glucose level will usually stay in the target range.

Just because you are going to count carbohydrates does not mean you can't eat them!

In fact, if you eat a well-balanced diet, half the calories you eat (45–55%) will come from carbs. Protein provides about 15% to 20% of the total calories while fats provide 30–35% or less.

For e.g.-If your daily meal plan contains 1,200 calories, about 600 (1/2 of the calories) will come from carbs.

Too much carbohydrates in one meal can make your blood glucose levels stay high for too long. Counting carbohydrates is one of the best and easiest ways to plan your meals and keep a check on your blood glucose levels. It provides an accurate estimate of how your blood glucose levels will rise after a meal or snack. Counting carbs can offer more variety to your meal plan.

You can learn to use carbohydrate counting to choose what and how much to eat. If you take insulin, you can use carbohydrate counting to decide how much insulin to take. One word of caution here is that you need to choose the right types of carbs as meals rich in simple carbs (bad carbs such as sugar, refined foods) and fat can cause your blood fats to get deranged leading to insulin resistance (obesity) and call for an increased requirement of insulin. The type and amount of carbs you eat is very important in ensuring that blood glucose and cholesterol levels are well within the target range.

Within your daily carbohydrate budget, it is recommended that you include foods providing good carbs such as unpolished cereals, pulses, sprouts, whole fruits, vegetables, and low-fat dairy products. Make an effort to include fibre rich foods like vegetables, fruits, whole grains and pulses as they aid in better blood glucose control.

Which foods have carbs?

- Grains – Bread, pasta, breakfast cereals, chapattis, rice, rice flakes, noodles, Semolina (rawa), Refined Flour (maida), Broken wheat (daliya), Oats, Sago (sabudana)
- Fruits and dried fruits
- Pulses – sprouts, dals, soya
- Vegetables especially roots and tubers-potato, sweet potato, tapioca, yam (suran), taro root (arbi), peas
- Milk and Milk products
- Sugar, honey and jaggery
- Desserts

Each of the foods below represent 15 g of carbohydrates

Food groups	Amount (g)	Household measure
Cereals (flours)	23	1/3rd cup
Rice flakes	20	1/3rd cup
Semolina (rawa)	20	1/4th cup
Pasta, Noodles	70	1 cup (cooked)
Bread/Pav	30	1.5 regular slices/1 no.
Pulse/Dal	30	1 palmful
Soyabean	150	1 cup
Soya granules	50	1 palmful
Elaichi Banana, Chickoo	65	1 no.
Pear, Apple	180/100	1 medium
Pomegranate/Papaya,	130/208	1 small/quarter plate
Orange, sweet limes	180/300	2 medium
Root vegetables (potato, suran)	100	1 medium/1/2 no.
Peas	130	3/4 cup
Buffalo Milk/Cow's Milk	180 ml/300 ml	1.2 cups/2 cups
Paneer	125	6 medium pcs
Curd	375	1.5 big cups

None or negligible Carbs (0–5 g carbs)

All vegetables (except root vegetables)

- Green leafy vegetable
- Nuts
- Spices
- Eggs

- Seafood
- Meat and poultry
- Fats (oil, butter and ghee)

How Do You Count Carbs?

The amount of carbohydrate you eat can make a big difference to your blood glucose levels. If you eat more carbohydrate than usual at a meal, your blood glucose level is likely to be higher than usual for up to several hours afterwards.

Carbohydrates are measured in grams and may be referred to in grams or 'servings'. One carbohydrate serving equals 15 grams of carbohydrate (1 carb serving=15 grams of carbohydrate). Sugar and foods that are almost pure sugar – a lollipop, candy, jaggery and honey – are easy to figure out. 15 grams of table sugar is 15 grams of carbohydrate – as simple as that.

You can check serving sizes with measuring cups, spoons or a food scale. Measuring food may seem difficult or annoying in the beginning, but it is very important. Once you do this exercise, you will be able to tell the carbs in the food without batting an eyelid. There are various apps available today which can give you the carbohydrate count of various foods.

> You can refer to the Nutrition Basics and Guide to Carbohydrate counting book authored by Sheryl Salis or download our app NHS-INC (Indian Nutrient Counter) from Google play store where you can get the nutrition values of more than 5000 foods.

For packaged foods, the easiest way is to read the nutrition facts section on the package. How to read a food label is covered in detail in the chapter on food labels.

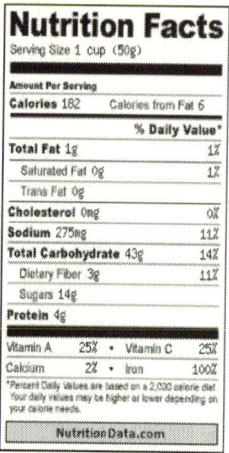

How to Count CHO Servings	
0-5gms	free food (do not count)
6-10gms	½
11-20gms	1
21-25gm	1 ½
26-35gms	2
45gms	3
60gms	4

Real life example

Ritu (name changed) is 22 years old and has diabetes for the past 3 years. She is a foodie and loves to experiment with food. She usually has a variety of foods for breakfast like poha, upma, idli, dosa, utappam, etc. She was bored of eating the same breakfast daily, so she decided to have only eggs and fruit for breakfast one day. She took her regular insulin shot and left for office. On her way, she started feeling symptoms of hypoglycaemia. On checking, she found that her blood glucose levels were 52mg/dl (2.9 mmol/l). She was confused as to why her glucose levels dropped in spite of having regular insulin and no extra exercise.

The reason why she encountered a hypo was that she did not count the carbs of her food. Every day for breakfast, she had food options which contained more carbs, but today she had eggs which have no carbs and fruit which had just 10 g carbs, hence the insulin requirement was much less. She had taken her regular insulin dose because of which her blood glucose levels dropped.

How Many Servings of Carbs Should You Eat at Each Meal?

The amount of carbohydrate will vary based on the needs of each individual. The recommended number of servings is based on your weight, activity level, diabetes medications, type of insulin and the goals set for your blood glucose levels. For many people, having 45–60 g of carbohydrate foods at each meal and 15-30 g for snacks works well. For children and adolescents it could be slightly different. Younger school-age children will consume 30–60 g of carbohydrate per meal, and older children and adolescents may consume up to 60–90 g of carbohydrate per meal. Older children who are more physically active will require more carbohydrate amounts than younger or less active children. Most children also consume 15–30 g of carbohydrate as between-meal snacks.

Depending on the type of insulin you are on, mid-meal snacks and bedtime milk may or may not be necessary. If you are on a fixed dose of insulin, you will need to keep the prescribed amount of carbohydrate more consistent at meals and snacks from day-to-day.

How much insulin you need to balance out a given amount of carbohydrate is determined by your carbohydrate to insulin ratio. For those on multiple-dose insulin therapy, taking rapid-acting or short-acting insulin before meals can use the insulin to carb ratio to match your insulin dosage to the amount of carbs you eat. This provides a great deal of flexibility to meal planning while helping you maintain your blood glucose in the optimal range.

For people with Type 2 diabetes, keeping a check on your carbs is extremely useful to help you control your weight and 'even out' your carbohydrate intake throughout the day. The beauty of carbohydrate counting is that your choice of what to eat at each meal is unlimited! All you have to do is make sure the carbohydrate count of your meal hits the target your dietitian recommends. You still need to be watchful of the quality of carbs you eat while keeping the quantity in check.

Insulin to Carb ratio

Dietary regulation and lack of dietary freedom are often reported by adolescents to be among the worst aspects of living with diabetes, and so dietary advice is often ignored. Counting carbs may improve compliance to treatment because it allows for flexibility in food choices. Carbohydrate counting is one of the tools that may empower children and adolescents to manage their own diabetes more effectively within their own lifestyle.

For those who think it's complicated, mind you, we have our young tots who have mastered the art and have become experts at carb counting.

Insulin: Carbohydrate ratio theory

The theory behind insulin: Carb (I:C) ratio is based on the assumption that the carbohydrates we eat from food are mostly responsible for raising blood glucose levels after meals. Fats and protein have a minimal effect on blood glucose levels particularly when consumed in small amounts (less than 20–30 g) as a part of a carbohydrate-rich meal.

As we are aware, rapid-acting or short-acting insulins are recommended to be taken at mealtimes (always before meals) and are responsible for controlling post-meal glucose spikes caused by the carbs in the meal we eat. For some adults, one unit of fast-acting insulin can usually cover 15 grams of carbohydrate, however, for a very young child, as little as 0.5 unit of fast-acting insulin might cover 15 grams of carbohydrate.

I:C ratio is the amount of carbs (grams) covered by one unit of insulin. Insulin to carb ratio will vary depending on the body weight, physical activity, insulin sensitivity and may be different at different times of the day. More the body weight, more insulin is required for a given amount of carbohydrates and higher the insulin sensitivity, less insulin is required for a given amount of carbohydrates.

I:C ratio gives you the flexibility to eat as much or as little carbohydrate as you choose while still maintaining good blood glucose control. I:C ratios will vary at different times of the day due to changes in hormone levels (which affect insulin sensitivity), physical activity (which enhances insulin sensitivity) and the amount of basal/long-acting insulin overlapping with the mealtime insulin.

It is important to calculate and set a specific ratio between carbohydrate amount and insulin dose for each individual.

One word of caution before we start is "Do not go too aggressive on the starting dose." It is best to begin with a lower insulin dose in order to prevent a hypoglycemic episode. We can always fine-tune the dose later rather than try adjusting when you're constantly recovering from low blood glucose levels.

There are two methods of calculating the I:C ratio

The 450/500 Rule

This approach is based on the assumption that on an average an individual consumes (via meals and snacks) and produces (via the liver) a total of approximately 500 grams of carbohydrate daily. By dividing 500 by the average number of units of insulin you take daily (total daily dose which is a sum of rapid-acting/bolus insulin and long-acting/basal insulin), you can get a reasonable approximation of your I:C ratio.

For example, if you take 5 units of rapid-acting insulin three times a day and 10 units of long-acting insulin once a day, the total daily dose (TDD) is 25 units.

500/TDD = 500/25 = 20

I:C ratio = 1:20 means each unit will cover 20 g of carbs.

A 30 g snack will need 1.5 units considering the 1:20 ratio

For people on regular/short-acting insulin we use the 450 rule

Divide 450 by the total daily dose of insulin to get an estimate of the grams of carbohydrate that is approximately covered by 1 unit of insulin.

For example, if TDD is 30 Units/day

450/30 = 15

1 unit of insulin covers 15 g of carbohydrate.

Example (Breakfast):

3 Toast: 30 g

Egg: 0 g

100 ml cow's Milk: 5 g

1 Apple: 15 g

Total Carbs: 50 g

Insulin to Carb Ratio 1:15

Amount of insulin required for this meal: 3.3 U

For very young children (less than 5 years) who need less than 10 units of insulin a day, the 300–350 rule is applicable instead of the 450/500 rule. In practice, the detailed records of self-monitored blood glucose (SMBG results), continuous glucose monitoring (CGM), carb intake and insulin doses provide useful information for making ratio adjustments.

Arriving at the right I:C ratio

An important note to be kept in mind when you begin using carb counting is that you will not get the right I:C ratio on day one. It will take several days and require constant fine-tuning by trial and error to arrive at the right I:C ratio. You should verify the I:C ratio at each meal and snack as they may vary at different times of the day.

For most people, insulin sensitivity tends to be a bit lower in the morning than later in the day due to the hormonal surge/dawn phenomena. For example, an individual may require a 1:10 ratio at breakfast, 1:12 at lunch, and 1:15 at dinner and in the evening, but if you exercise in the evening, the I:C ratio may even drop to 1:25.

In the case of children, the I:C ratio is usually highest in the morning, lower for lunch and higher in the evening. The amount of activity and energy requirements in children changes very frequently. Therefore, the variability of the ICR in children is usually much larger than that of adults.

As the second number in the ratio goes up, the amount of insulin required goes down.

Real life example

Bhushan (name changed) has diabetes and is dependent on insulin. He has learnt to count carbs and takes his insulin dosage after counting the carbs in every meal. He takes his insulin dose after the meal. In spite of counting carbs, his HbA1c was 8.1. After consulting me, he realized that though he was counting carbs, he did not check his blood glucose levels frequently so he did not have a clue of how the food was affecting his blood glucose level.

Since he was on rapid-acting insulin, he was advised to take his insulin 10–15 minutes before the meal, check his blood glucose levels 2 hours after a meal especially when he introduced new food items in his menu. He started keeping a food log – food that he ate, insulin dose and glucose monitoring results. This started giving him an idea of how the sugars were responding to his insulin dosage.

After Bhushan started checking his blood glucose levels regularly, he realized that though he was counting carbohydrates correctly, his insulin to carb ratio required fine-tuning. After consulting the doctor and setting his insulin to carb ratios, his blood glucose levels started falling in the normal range and within 3 months, he achieved an HbA1c of 6.9%.

A Few Points to Remember When Calculating Insulin to Carb Ratio

- Verify the total daily dose every time you make a change in the basal or bolus insulin dose.

- Do not consider one day's insulin dosage. Take an average of the last 10–14 days total insulin units that were taken and consider the average total daily dose for calculation.

- Maintain a record in your diary of what you eat, the bolus (insulin for meals and correction dose) taken and other factors like stress, and physical activity when evaluating your I:C ratio.

- Make a note of all the blood glucose readings taken before and 2–4 hours after a meal. If the blood glucose levels after 2–4 hours are in the target range, this means that the I:C ratio set for this meal is right. Ensure that you do not eat, exercise or take another shot of insulin between the two blood glucose readings as they may affect the test results.

- It is best to eliminate factors other than food that might be affecting the results of the tests. For example, do not include data collected during or immediately after strenuous exercise. Most people find that their blood glucose levels are high post-exercise. It is recommended that you wait for at least half an hour post the activity before you test your blood glucose.

The I:C ratio which may be right for a meal today but may raise your blood glucose levels for the same meal tomorrow. This is because there are many external factors which influence the blood glucose readings. Be sure to rule out these factors when analysing the data.

- Weekday and Weekends
- Sleep pattern
- Eating out versus eating home-cooked meals
- Physical activity
- Menstruation
- Emotional and mental stress
- Illness
- Medication schedules
- High fat and protein (> 20 g fat and > 30 g protein per serving) meals
- A higher insulin dose (bolus as well as basal) may be required during this period.

In case of pump or insulin therapy, rule out the following factors:

- Insulin potency (if cold chain not maintained)
- Air bubble in the insulin reservoir resulting in a failed delivery
- Insulin vial/cartridge – syringe and vial used (40IU, 100IU)
- Day of change of the infusion set (recommended to be changed every three days)
- Insulin injection/infusion site (rotation of sites is a must to prevent lipoatrophy)

- Insulin stacking (taking insulin within a gap of 4–5 hours from the previous shot resulting in hypoglycaemia)

No/low Carb snacking options (do not need insulin if taken in limited amounts)

- Plain Yogurt/Curd
- Salted Buttermilk
- Handful of Unsalted Nuts and seeds (almonds, walnuts, pistachios, pumpkin seeds, sunflower seeds)
- Vegetable sticks (Raw carrot, beetroot, cucumber, celery stalks) with Hung Curd Dip
- Avocado/Guacamole Dip
- Cheese
- Cottage Cheese (paneer) – Grilled/Tikka/Vegetable
- Eggs (boiled, omelette, Spanish omelette, egg muffins, poached, scrambled)
- Egg/Chicken/Paneer Salad
- Peanuts (unsalted)
- Soy nuts
- Small portion of fruit
- Rasam/clear soups
- Sauted mushrooms

Fat and Protein Counting

Foods which contain a high amount of protein and fat along with carbohydrate take a longer time to digest causing the blood glucose levels to rise much later. Hence, it will be necessary to consider additional dosing of insulin for meals containing more than 20 g fat and 30 g protein. However, any changes in insulin dosing should be done under the supervision of your doctor as different people have different sensitivities to fat and protein.

Examples of food with more than 30 g protein

Food	Amount	Protein
Non-veg Burger	1 no.	30–50 g
Chicken (leg pc)	3 no.	30 g
Fish	3 medium pc (> 125 g)	25–30 g
Non-veg pizza	3–4 slices	30–40 g
Chicken/Mutton curry	1 soup bowl (6–7 pcs chicken/mutton)	30–40 g
Paneer	150 g	30 g
Cheese	130 g (5 cheese cubes)	30–35 g
Soybean	80 g	30 g
Soy Chunks	70 g	35 g

For only protein meals with less than 75 g protein, additional insulin dose may not be required.

Examples of food with > 20 g fat

Food	Amount	Fat
French fries	150 g (Medium Size)	25 g
Cheese cake/slice cake/muffins	Single pc	20–30 g
Creamy pasta in white sauce/lasagne	Large Serving	20–40 g
Pizza (12")	3 slices	30 g
Burger	1 no.	20–65 g

Disclaimer: These are average values of nutrients and may vary based on the method of preparation and ingredients.

Insulin Sensitivity Factor

The insulin sensitivity factor (ISF) is defined as the amount of blood glucose (mg/dl) reduced by a unit of rapid or short-acting insulin. The 1800 rule and 1500rule are commonly accepted as the formulas for determining ISF. The rules calculate ISF by dividing either 1800 or 1500 by the total daily insulin dose. The 1800 rule is used for rapid-acting insulin and the 1500 rule for short-acting insulin. You can take the help of a qualified dietitian to know your I:C and ISF ratio.

Calculation of ISF (Sensitivity factor): 1800 Rule

1800 ÷ TDD (basal+ bolus) = ISF

If total daily dose (TDD) is 60, then

Insulin sensitivity factor is = 1800/TDD

= 1800/60

= 30

That means 1 unit of insulin will drop your glucose levels by 30 mg/dl ((1.7mmol/l)

The values calculated by these formulas are just starting points. Frequent blood glucose monitoring will be needed to calculate the actual ISF. Just as with I:C ratio, ISF may change daily as well at different times within the same day.

For example, ISF may be 50 mg/dl(2.8 mmol/l) in the morning, 70 mg/dl (3.9mmol/l) at lunch, and 60 mg/dl (3.3mmol/l) in the evening. For infants and toddlers, ISF is higher, almost 100–150 mg/dl. The fluctuation of ISF in children is usually greater than that of an adult. Therefore, a record of self-monitoring of blood glucose (SMBG) results, carb intake, impact of physical activity and insulin doses, need to be maintained and reviewed on a regular basis.

Don't give up when you don't get it right the first few times. It is a learning process and will need constant fine-tuning before you get it perfect. Don't let the 'one off' odd reading bother and de-motivate you. The key is to look for trends and patterns in your data. If your blood glucose levels are in the steady range on most occasions, this means the I:C ratio and ISF set are right for you.

One word of caution during carb counting is that one tends to ignore the principles of good nutrition as they focus only on the carb content of the meal without paying much attention to the protein and fat content of the meal. By doing this, you may end up consuming a diet low in protein and high in fat leading to weight gain, muscle loss and an increased risk of heart disease. Weight gain will further cause insulin resistance resulting in an increased requirement of insulin.

Also, once an individual has mastered the art of carb counting, one tends to think that it is not necessary to consult a doctor/diabetes educator. This is where one falters.

Real life example

Adar (name changed) was a 16 year old school going boy (in Std X) from an affluent family, on insulin pump therapy with a total daily dose of 116 units. He skipped breakfast most days and ate most of his meals from out as he did not like the food cooked at home. He had not visited his doctor for more than a year, wasn't monitoring his blood glucose levels in the last one year. His family was shocked to see his HbA1c had shot up to 13.2%. They came to me for a consultation.

Height: 165 cm

Weight: 62 Kg

FBS: 280 mg/dl (15.5mmol/l)

PPBS: 356 mg/dl (19.8 mmol/l)

HbA1c: 13.2%

Wake up-6.00 A.M.

School-7 A.M. to 3.00 P.M.

Non-vegetarian

Diet Recall
<u>7.00 A.M.</u> A glass of Milk
<u>10.30 A.M. Breakfast</u> (In school break)- 2nd break –
<u>3.30.P.M. Lunch</u> Burgers OR Pizza
<u>6.00 P.M. Evening</u> Biscuits/Chips/Vadas/Samosas
<u>9.30 P.M. Dinner</u> Restaurant food Chicken Biryani/Chicken Lollipops/Tawa Pulao/Fried Rice/Manchurian
I counselled the family on the importance of following a disciplined lifestyle and importance of monitoring. He assured me that he will give his best shot to bring down his blood glucose levels by eating healthy and indulging in regular physical activity
Diet Planned
Before going to school – A glass of milk with handful of nuts

10.30 A.M. Breakfast (In school break)
Egg Wrap(with vegetables)/Muesli (No sugar)/Oats with milk/Sprouts

2nd break
Fruit (1 portion)

3.30.P.M. Lunch
Salad
Buttermilk
Chapatti/Rice
Dal/Chicken

6.00 P.M. Evening
Egg/chicken/egg/paneer (warm) Salad/Wrap/Roasted Makhana/Moong/ Besan Chilla

9.30 P.M. Dinner
Salad
Vegetable
Chicken Curry/Fish Curry/Dal
Chapatti/Rice

He started monitoring more often, put a continuous glucose monitor (CGM) on and started swimming and walking regularly. He would report daily. He started feeling more energetic than before and could concentrate on his studies better.

His parents were very happy to see that in less than six months, his insulin dose came down by half from 116 U to 60 U and HbA1c dropped from 13.2 % to 7.1%. His fasting blood glucose levels were between 100mg/dl to 120 mg/dl and post meals between 130mg/dl (7.2mmol/l) and 150 mg/dl (8.3mmol/l) on most days. His CGMS showed his blood glucose readings were in the desired range more than 75% of the time (Time in range). He did not experience any high or low blood glucose levels.

Remember there's more to diabetes management than just managing blood glucose levels make sure you get your doctor, diabetes educator to review your data and give you feedback from time to time. My patients usually like to review their readings with me over a personal consultation, phone, email to get a reassurance that they are on the right track.

CHAPTER 10 Hypoglycaemia

Low blood glucose levels!! While this may be the best news for some people whose blood glucose levels are always high, this is not what we health professionals like.

Low blood glucose is also known as hypoglycaemia (hypo-low, glycaemia – glucose in the blood). People with diabetes usually on insulin and other diabetes medications are at risk of hypoglycaemia. It is a more dangerous situation than high blood glucose and needs to be treated immediately.

Reasons for hypoglycaemia or low blood glucose can be many. Skipping a meal or eating too little and taking too much insulin or tablets, exercise, extra activity (cleaning the house), taking a hot shower immediately after an insulin injection, alcohol – all these factors can cause hypoglycaemia.

Real life example

Akash (name changed) is 44 years old with very poor blood glucose control. The doctor suggested insulin regime to help him get his glucose levels in the normal range. After starting the insulin, he used to feel dizzy and hungry within a few hours of taking the insulin shot in spite of having his regular meals. He came to me for nutrition guidance as his post-meals blood glucose levels were going very low and he was constantly hungry. He came to my clinic with his insulin syringe and vial. The vial he was using was a 100 IU vial and the syringe was 40 IU. This means he was taking 2.5 times extra insulin because of which he was recurrently going into hypoglycaemia after his meals and was also feeling very hungry.

It is very important to buy the right IU vial and syringe. If you are using a 40 IU vial, always use a 40 IU syringe (red cap, red markings on the syringe). Once he changed the syringe that he was using, his blood glucose levels started falling in the normal range. His constant feeling of hunger which was related to his low blood glucose levels also disappeared.

Another real life example

Kirti (name changed) is 9 years old with type1 diabetes. She was on multiple injections of insulin regime and always experienced low blood glucose episodes after her meal. In spite of reducing the doses her hypoglycaemia was becoming difficult to handle. She came to me for her nutrition consultation. On investigating further, I realized that she was very lean and thin with very little subcutaneous fat. She injected insulin 90 degrees straight on the thigh, which means she was injecting in the muscle which caused rapid absorption of glucose leading to hypoglycaemia. When I advised her on the right technique and the right site to take the insulin shot, the hypo-episodes reduced considerably.

Common mistakes which can cause hypoglycaemia

People with diabetes who are on the insulin injection regime have a higher chance of developing hypoglycaemia. Many children with diabetes experience hypoglycaemia as their parents are busy chasing numbers. The fear of being shouted at for high blood glucose levels compels them to inject more insulin on the sly and this results in hypoglycaemia.

Also, some children who are very active inject insulin on the thigh and start running around which increases the absorption of insulin due to exercise. It is recommended to check with your doctor the site to inject insulin.

Another common mistake is that people take all their medications at one go, instead of taking it at the times prescribed by the doctor. Certain anti-diabetes medications act in such a way that they stimulate your pancreas to secrete more insulin. If you take these medications and miss a meal or eat later, you may be at risk of hypoglycaemia. Hypoglycaemia caused by these medications can be more prolonged and last for up to 24 to 48 hours. Hypoglycaemia can be caused due to various reasons but it is important to identify the underlying cause of hypoglycaemia and correct that instead of just treating hypoglycaemia alone.

Depending on the severity, hypoglycaemia reactions can be of three types – mild, moderate and severe.

The symptoms of mild hypoglycaemia include nervousness, shakiness, palpitations (rapid heartbeat), sweating, dizziness, yawning, weakness, blurred vision, headache and hunger. Never ignore these symptoms. Hypoglycaemia is always a medical emergency, and you have to take care of it on priority! It is important to always carry glucose tablets or keep glucose-containing foods handy to avoid and treat any hypo-emergencies.

When having symptoms, always check blood glucose levels first to ensure if it is actually below the normal range (which is 70 mg/dl or 3.9 mmol/l).

You can immediately correct a hypo by taking any kind of a fast-acting carbohydrate source: Glucose tablets or gels, 3 teaspoons of glucose or sugar (glucose is preferred), fruit juice, a regular soft drink (with sugar – not sugar-free), candy/lozenges, glucose tablets, anything you can get your hands on.

Repeat blood glucose testing after 15 minutes and continue treatment until the blood glucose level returns to the normal range. After correcting your blood glucose level, it is recommended to have at least a 15 g carb snack with protein like a paneer wrap or an egg wrap (multigrain/whole wheat roti), fruits with nuts to avoid further hypoglycaemia episodes. The amount of fast-acting carbs/glucose you take will depend on the blood glucose level, body size and rate of blood glucose drop. For younger children the amount of glucose to correct a hypoglycaemia could be lower. Speak to your doctor and dietitian to know the amount of simple fast-acting carbs you need to take during a hypo-episode.

Real life example

Sai (name changed) is an MBA student and has diabetes. He used to spend long hours in college. Whenever he experienced a hypo-symptom, he would rush to the college canteen and have a tetra pack of mango juice with fried snacks available as he used to be ravenously hungry. He loved these hypo-episodes as it gave him an opportunity to have his favourite foods. But later when he became vigilant about his blood glucose, he realised that after every episode of hypo, his blood glucose levels spiked up to 300–350 mg/dl (16.7–19.4mmol/l)

This is a very common example of hypo-over correction.

Whenever the blood glucose levels are low, your body needs approx. 15 g of simple carbohydrate to raise the level. If you look at the food label on these juice packs, most of these juices approx. 100 ml have about 13.5 g of carbohydrates. If you drink a glass of juice i.e. 200 ml the carbohydrate content in your juice is 2 x 13.5 = 27 g and if you drink the entire pack of juice it is still higher.

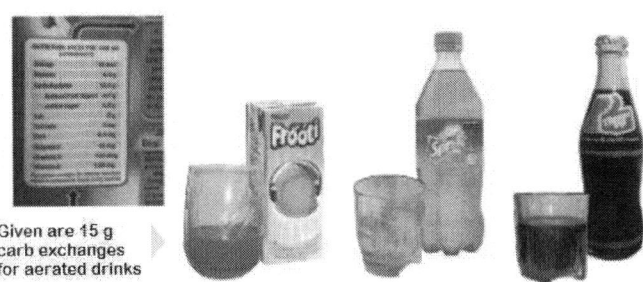

Given are 15 g carb exchanges for aerated drinks

As juice is direct sugar and it raises your blood glucose levels rapidly, I advised Sai to have just half a glass of juice during hypo or a better option is to keep glucose tablets with him in his bag.

Just by following the guidelines given, Sai was able to avoid the yo-yo effect of hypoglycaemia.

Real life example

Diti (name changed) is a sportsperson and is very active during the day. Though her doses are adjusted keeping in mind her schedules, there are times when she faces hypo-every time she changes her fitness routine.

Diti had a sweet tooth and whenever she was in a hypo-state she would eat anything sweet that came her way. She could not control her cravings and her hunger pangs during the hypo-episode and would end up eating biscuits, pastries, chocolates or even junk food. After that she would take a correction dose for all the extra food that she had. Most of the time, she would overcorrect herself to avoid high blood glucose levels leading to another hypo-episode.

I explained to Diti the rule of 15–15 i.e. have 15 g or 3 tsp of glucose/sugar mixed well with water and check your sugars after 15 minutes. If it is still low, she can correct with 15 g of glucose/sugar again. Once the blood glucose level reaches the normal levels, it is necessary to have 15 g carbs with protein meal to sustain the sugar levels. Having a carb and protein combination works best as an after hypo-meal. You can eat a paneer wrap or egg wrap or chapatti and cheese, have fruits and nuts etc. Do not gulp it down. Eat mindfully taking small bites. Relish each small bite and as the sugar comes in the normal range, the urge to binge diminishes.

Biscuits, pastries, Indian high-fat sweets and chocolates are not recommended as they are high in fat and tend to raise blood glucose levels after 3–4 hours and not immediately. Hence, it is advisable not to eat anything high in fat while treating a hypo-episode.

Deciphering hypoglycaemia in a better way

The standard recommendation to manage a hypo-episode is to always test when you feel low. This will confirm that your blood glucose levels are really low. Symptoms of hypoglycaemia are sometimes similar to hyperglycaemia (high blood glucose). If you do not have a blood glucose monitor with you, treat yourself thinking your blood glucose levels are low. Remember hypoglycaemia can be more serious and dangerous than hyperglycaemia.

If low, take 15 grams of carbohydrate (3 tsp of glucose/sugar in water or 4 glucose tablets). If mixing sugar in water, remember to stir well till the sugar dissolves. You can add a pinch of salt so that the absorption of glucose is faster.

Test again after 15 minutes, if still low take another 15 grams of carbohydrate. Never leave home without carrying your ID card and sugar sachets/glucose tabs/dry fruits like dates/figs/raisins or a few candies in your handbag.

If left untreated, hypoglycaemia can get progressively worse and leave you less and less able to help yourself. Without a quick dose of fast-acting carbohydrate, your hypoglycaemia may progress to what is called "moderate hypoglycaemia" – although those who have experienced it say there is nothing "moderate" about it. Symptoms of moderate hypoglycaemia include confusion, poor coordination, inability to cooperate, and slurred speech.

In the first stages of moderate hypoglycaemia, you may still be able to help yourself by drinking some juice or eating some candy. But as it advances you may have to rely on someone else to squirt a tube of icing sugar or glucose gels between your gum and cheek as you may no longer be in a state of full consciousness. After the icing sugar takes effect, you should have a substantial carb and protein combined snack.

Severe Hypoglycaemia

The most serious kind of hypoglycaemia is 'severe hypoglycaemia,' characterized by unresponsiveness, unconsciousness or convulsions. If severe hypoglycaemia strikes, you are powerless to help yourself and require assistance from another individual for appropriate treatment. Please let your relatives/caregivers know that they should not try and give you anything orally (by mouth) as it could lead to aspiration and choking. However they can try making a paste of glucose and water and rubbing the same on the inside of the cheek.

You are encouraged to keep glucagon injections at home which can be injected in the muscle to treat severe hypoglycaemia, even by family members. Nowadays glucagon inhalers are also available. Speak to your doctor to know more details about it.

If glucagon is not available, it is best to be taken to the hospital casualty for intravenous glucose. If you/your child are required to be given glucagon, it is essential to check blood glucose levels 2 and 4 hours later, as there is a risk of the blood glucose level going low at that time again.

Real life example

Niyati (name changed) has diabetes and is a very active person. Whenever she would experience a bout of hypo, she would avoid eating sugar and would instead treat it with mithais or biscuits. During one such episode, like always she had biscuits to correct the blood glucose level and started doing her regular work. Within a few minutes, she started feeling dizzy and she fainted. Her family members rushed her to the hospital.

The doctors explained that she had fainted because of low blood glucose levels. The truth was that when she felt low, she corrected it with cream biscuits. Biscuits are made from refined flour or maida and fats hence it takes longer to get converted into sugar.

Hence it is always prudent to take simple and easily absorbable carbs like 3 teaspoons glucose/sugar or 3–4 glucose tablets and wait till the blood glucose level reaches the normal range. Only once the blood glucose levels have come to the normal range should you have something to eat, ideally food that has 15 grams carbohydrates.

Nocturnal hypoglycaemia (hypoglycaemia at night)

Nocturnal hypoglycaemia (hypoglycaemia at night) is a common problem and often goes unnoticed and undetected. It is important for the patient's partner to keep checking for symptoms such as profuse sweating, restlessness and convulsions. If you get up in the morning with a severe headache, have a hangover feeling or do not feel satisfied with the sleep (feel like you've not slept enough), find your pillow wet, chances are that you have gone low in the night.

When you check your blood glucose levels in the morning, in all probability, they will be high. This is a rebound effect on the low blood glucose episode. Sensing low blood glucose in the blood, the liver breaks down its glycogen stores and releases glucose in the blood resulting in high blood glucose levels. Based on this reading, you increase the night dose of insulin which may cause you to go into severe hypoglycaemia in the middle of the night and can even lead to a coma which can be life-threatening.

If you are on an intermediate-acting insulin (insulatard, huminsulin N, and any other NPH insulin brands) or on premix insulin 30/70 or 50/50, check blood glucose levels at bedtime and keep them above 100 to 140 mg/dl (5.6–7.8 mmol/l). On days of activity like physical training (PT) days in school or on days where you have exerted yourself more than usual, check your blood glucose level at bedtime and at 3 A.M. Aim for a 3 A.M. blood glucose level above 70 mg/dl (3.9 mmol/l). If blood glucose is repeatedly low at bedtime and 3 A.M., revise the insulin/tablet dose after you have consulted the doctor. Check blood glucose levels at 5 P.M. and aim at keeping it between 80 and 130 mg/dl (4.4–7.2 mmol/l). A blood glucose level at 5 P.M. below 80mg/dl indicates a high chance of blood glucose levels dropping at night.

Some of the recommended bedtime snacks are milk with nuts, date-chana/date nut roll which will keep the blood glucose levels sustained through the night.

Keep a blood glucose monitor, glucose tablets/sachets and water at your bedside always. Patients on basal long-acting insulin and bolus rapid-acting insulin have lesser chances of hypoglycaemia. They may not require taking a bedtime snack. It is important to speak to your diabetes educator about this.

Hypoglycaemia Unawareness

There is a condition called hypoglycaemia unawareness which means you do not experience any symptoms of hypoglycaemia and go unconscious without realizing what is happening to you. This is often seen in adults and children where, because of repeated hypoglycaemia, the body becomes used to it and does not sense the blood glucose levels dropping. Elderly people or people with long-standing diabetes are also at risk as they have neuropathy (a complication where the nerves are affected in diabetes) and fail to give out signals of low blood glucose. This can be very detrimental and dangerous.

Blood glucose targets need to be revised and kept higher for people who go into recurrent hypoglycaemia at night, especially elderly people and children who have hypoglycaemia unawareness. Review your medication and blood glucose readings with your doctor and set your blood glucose goals. Speak to your doctor about the continuous blood glucose monitoring sensor (CGMS) or the ambulatory blood glucose profile (AGP) which gives you a complete picture of your blood glucose trends over 6 to 14 days. This will give you a better idea of your blood glucose trends and the action that needs to be taken.

A fruit parfait is a perfect to be had after correcting a hypo-episode with glucose.

Fruit Parfait

Ingredients

1 handful of chopped strawberries, ½ cup hung curd, a handful of crushed nuts

Method

Place the chopped strawberries in a glass jar. Layer it with hung curd. Add some crushed nuts of your choice and your fruit parfait is ready.

This can be had instead of the flavoured fruits yogurt that is available in the supermarket which is loaded with sugar.

Key Takeaway

Hypoglycaemia is serious – and it should be taken seriously!! Your best defence is to monitor your blood glucose frequently, carefully balance your insulin and medication with your food intake, always keep some fast-acting sugar at hand – and act immediately when you feel the symptoms of hypoglycaemia setting in. Always carry your diabetes identity card with you.

Sick Days

A 13-year-old girl with a known case of type 1 diabetes developed cold and cough due to change in weather. Her blood glucose level was shooting up and hence her mother called me to know what to do as her doctor was out of town.

Fasting Blood Glucose: 295 mg/dl (16.4 mmol/l)

Postprandial Blood Glucose: 399 mg/dl (22.17 mmol/l)

Medications:

Rapid-Acting: 4U – 6U – 5U

Long-Acting: 0–0-10U

She was also on antibiotics for upper respiratory tract infection.

The child had a very severe respiratory tract infection due to which she wasn't able to eat much. Because her intake of food was so little, her mother was not giving insulin. I explained to the mother on the importance of taking insulin during sick days. Since she is feeling too sick to eat, the body will get its energy by releasing blood glucose from stored supplies in the liver, making blood glucose level rise further. That is why taking insulin when sick, to control blood glucose levels becomes extremely important. I told her to ask her doctor on the insulin dose to give.

Due to her health condition, the child found it difficult to swallow food. I asked the mother to give her soft foods like porridge, khichdi, fruit as her regular foods to equal the amount of carbohydrates that she would normally eat.

I also asked her to monitor her blood glucose levels and ketones, every 4 hours.

If blood glucose is over 250 mg/dl (13.9 mmol/l), I advised her to drink any one of the below options

- Water (with lime and salt)
- Soups or vegetable juices
- Salted buttermilk

She followed the advice and started taking insulin as recommended by her doctor. Her blood glucose levels came within the normal range.

CHAPTER 11
Gestational Diabetes Mellitus (GDM)

We all know about Type 1 and Type 2 diabetes, but there is another type of diabetes that not many know about. This type of diabetes occurs in pregnant women and is known as Gestational Diabetes Mellitus or GDM. It occurs during pregnancy, or is first discovered during pregnancy usually during the second or third trimester.

Pregnancy results in many changes in body functions and may affect the way the body controls blood glucose levels. Gestational diabetes can occur as a result of hormonal changes a pregnant woman's body experiences. During pregnancy, the placenta produces hormones that interfere with the action of insulin, the hormone that regulates blood glucose. In a normal pregnancy, the woman's pancreas compensates for this by making additional insulin. If your body is not able to meet the increased demand for insulin during pregnancy, blood glucose levels rise resulting in gestational diabetes (GDM).

In most women, GDM disappears once the baby is born.

How does GDM affect you or your baby?

Most women with gestational diabetes have healthy pregnancies and healthy babies. Early diagnosis, right treatment and frequent monitoring can ensure a healthy pregnancy and its outcome. However if blood glucose levels are not controlled, GDM increases certain risks for the mother and baby.

Possible risks for the mother include:

- Higher chance of needing a C-section
- Miscarriage
- High blood pressure or preeclampsia

Mothers with GDM have a risk of developing GDM in the next pregnancy and 50% chance of developing type 2 diabetes mellitus (T2DM) within 20 years following their diagnosis of GDM.

Possible risks for the baby include:

- Injuries during delivery because of the baby's size

  If your blood glucose level is high, there is increased glucose delivery to the baby, which forces the baby's pancreas to produce more insulin. This causes the baby to grow large which might cause issues in a normal delivery.

- Low blood glucose and mineral levels at birth
- Jaundice, a treatable condition that makes the skin yellowish
- Pre-term birth
- Temporary breathing problems
- Higher risk to obesity and diabetes in later life.

So after your delivery, ensure that you and your child follow a healthy lifestyle to lower the risk of developing lifestyle diseases later in life.

Keep in mind that just because you have gestational diabetes does not mean that these problems will occur.

What extra care do I need to take during pregnancy?

Care has to be taken towards keeping your blood glucose levels in the target range. Controlling your blood glucose is the key to preventing problems during pregnancy or birth. Your doctor will help you set your targets.

The key factors which will help you manage your blood glucose levels include:

- Healthy eating
- Physical activity
- Regular monitoring
- Insulin injections/Oral medications, if needed.

Healthy eating

You can take your dietitian's help to choose foods wisely that will provide the necessary nutrition for you and your baby, and that at the same time will not cause blood glucose levels to spike. A balanced, moderate carbohydrate, adequate protein, healthy fat and high fibre diet will ensure a healthy pregnancy and baby. This kind of a healthy diet is good for you to follow throughout pregnancy and after, as you raise your family. You can read more about GDM and dietary guidelines in the section ahead.

Physical activity

Along with dietary modifications, exercise has a very important role to play in maintaining blood glucose targets. Being physically active reduces your risk to develop type 2 diabetes in the future. Talk to your doctor about which activity is best suited for you.

- Aim for at least 30 minutes of exercise daily.
- Do aerobic activities like walking, swimming or low-impact aerobics.
- Choose an activity which is enjoyable and safe at the same time with minimum risk to injury or falls.

Regular self-monitoring

This is a very important part of managing GDM and is in your hands. Regular glucose monitoring can help you to understand how well you are responding to diet, exercise and treatment and can help your doctor to regulate the treatment more effectively. A detailed description on the importance of monitoring, how often and how you should monitor is given in the section ahead.

Insulin/Medications

If you have trouble meeting your blood glucose targets by dietary modifications and physical activity alone, you may need to take medication or insulin injections, along with following a healthy meal plan and being physically active. These insulin injections or oral medications need to be taken only till the pregnancy lasts and will stop once you deliver and your blood glucose is back to normal.

The first step in treating gestational diabetes is to modify your diet to help keep your blood glucose level in the normal range, while still eating a healthy balanced diet. Most women with well controlled blood glucose levels deliver healthy babies without any complications.

What diet should I follow if I have GDM?

When one is diagnosed with diabetes during pregnancy or gestational diabetes (GDM) there is often a fear associated with food. You may be constantly worried about what to eat as your doctor will emphasize on tight blood glucose control. Although foods have a direct impact on post-meal blood glucose levels, eating the right food in controlled portions can help in keeping your blood glucose levels in the normal range. The main aim of managing gestational diabetes is ensuring that your blood glucose levels are under control while making sure that you are providing adequate nourishment to yourself and your baby.

The good news is that you will be able to keep your blood glucose levels under control by changing what you eat and combining your new healthy diet with regular exercise. A GDM diet is simply a healthy balanced diet, timely placed with emphasis on portion control along with improving protein, calcium, iron and fibre intake and reducing refined foods. This will help control your blood glucose levels, provide adequate nutrition to you and your baby and prevent excessive weight gain during pregnancy.

Carbohydrates: The biggest challenge in pregnancy is high post-meal blood glucose levels. Usually the fasting blood glucose levels are in the desired range. Measuring and controlling post-meal glucose levels is critical during gestational diabetes. One way of keeping your blood glucose levels in the normal range is by monitoring the amount of carbohydrates in your diet.

Carbohydrates have the greatest impact on your blood glucose levels. They get converted to glucose within the first two hours of eating. The quantity, quality and distribution of carbohydrates throughout the day affects blood glucose control. Choosing the right type and amount (50% of total calories) of carbohydrate is very important in maintaining glucose levels in the target range.

The glycemic index (GI) (as mentioned in the chapter on glycemic index) of a food refers to the speed with which the food raises blood glucose levels. While all carbohydrates (except for fibre) convert into glucose eventually; some convert much faster than others.

Complex carbohydrates which are low GI like vegetables, whole fruits (apple, orange, pears, peach etc.), whole pulses and sprouts – kidney beans, black eyed beans, soybeans, whole moong (green gram), whole cereal grains –whole wheat, brown rice, barley, buckwheat, rolled or steel-cut oats, pasta made from durum wheat or quinoa should be preferred over high GI foods like polished rice, bread, pasta, maida and its products, cornflakes, baked potato, sugary foods etc. Make sure you spread the carbohydrate intake throughout the day to avoid post-meal spikes in blood glucose.

Fibre: Include fibre in the diet to help keep yourself full longer, prevent constipation and stabilize blood glucose levels. Make sure to include whole fruits, vegetables (salads and unstrained soups), and sprouts in your daily diet.

Protein: Protein requirements increase in pregnancy as they are the building materials of the body responsible for growth, maintenance and energy. Proteins flatten the glucose response of the food i.e. reduces glycemic index of food. Protein sources like lean meat, sprouts, egg whites, low-fat milk, yoghurt, cottage cheese (paneer), dals/pulses and defatted soya should be consumed. Combination of cereals and pulses (e.g. dal khichdi) are a good source of protein. Avoid fish which tend to have a high level of mercury like shark and tuna. Avoid intake of shellfish, raw or uncooked eggs and unpasteurized milk to reduce risk of food poisoning.

Fat: The biggest myth during pregnancy is that increasing your intake of oil and ghee gives a bonny baby. The fact is that although some amount of fat is necessary, the excessive intake will result in weight gain, increased insulin requirements and worsening of blood glucose levels. Excessive weight gain also increases the risk of developing type 2 diabetes in the future. Limit total consumption of oil, ghee, and butter. Choose a diet low in saturated fat – choose low-fat dairy foods, leans meats, and de-skinned chicken. Avoid the intake of biscuits, chips, cakes, pastries, processed fried, samosas, wadas, khari, butter, Indian sweets, ready-to-eat and takeaway foods.

Include omega-3 fatty acid rich foods.

Calcium: Calcium requirements double up in pregnancy. Calcium-rich foods such as skimmed/toned milk, curd and paneer, cheese, fish, green leafy vegetables, sesame seeds (til), finger millet (ragi), amaranth (rajgira) must be included in the diet.

Include iron-rich sources like pearl millet (bajra), finger millet (ragi), kidney beans (rajma), soybean, turnip greens, and green leafy vegetables. Squeeze lime on food to enhance the iron absorption.

The following are a few dietary recommendations that will help you maintain safe blood glucose levels:

Distribute your foods between three meals and two or three low carb snacks each day.

Eating too much at one time can cause your blood glucose to rise rapidly. Eating three small – to moderate-sized meals and two to three snacks (low carbohydrate, high protein) per day is recommended to distribute carbohydrate intake and reduce postprandial glucose fluctuations.

It is very important that you do not skip meals. Remember that during pregnancy, you have increased nutritional needs and your baby requires balanced nutrition for optimum growth and development.

Real life example

Hetal (name changed) was diagnosed with diabetes in her third trimester. She lived in a joint family and her in-laws were very happy as they were expecting their first grandchild in the family. Her mother in law took good care of her. She cooked food that she liked and forced her to eat more thinking that she needs to eat for 2 people. She fed her extra rotis with ghee or made her eat at least 3–4 fruits each day. In the bargain, Hetal started putting on extra weight and her blood glucose levels were never in range.

Though it is true that you have increased nutritional needs and your baby requires balanced nutrition for optimum growth and development but it is important not to go overboard. It is a myth that a woman needs to eat for two people. In fact the caloric requirement increases by only 350 calories and protein by 23 g per day in pregnancy.

Eating extra meals would mean additional weight gain that could harm the baby.

In modern times, doctors recommend a weight gain of not more than 6 to 8 kg in the nine months of pregnancy most of which must be gained in the second and third trimester.

When Hetal visited me to understand her meal plan, I designed a new plan for her with a combination of healthy carbs, protein, fat and fibre which helped her manage her blood glucose levels, kept her active and managed her weight at the same time.

By being disciplined towards her eating habits, Hetal managed her pregnancy and delivery beautifully.

Make wise breakfast choices and split the breakfast

Blood glucose can be difficult to control in the morning because of normal fluctuations in hormone levels.

Refined cereals and bread may cause your blood glucose levels to rise, hence are not a good choice for breakfast. Most women eat biscuits or toast as they experience morning sickness but this shoots up the blood glucose levels.

Remember, as the pregnancy progresses, insulin resistance increases and eating a high carbohydrate breakfast will cause the blood glucose levels to stay high throughout the day. It is thus advisable that the first meal is low in carbohydrates and high in protein to avoid the undue spikes in post-breakfast plasma glucose levels. An egg, a handful of nuts or a pulse based breakfast like moong khakra/moong dosa/moong chilla is the best choice for the first meal of the day followed by a low glycemic index low glycemic load meal at breakfast.

Drink one cup of milk at a time

Milk is an important source of protein and calcium and often recommended in pregnancy. However, milk is a liquid form of carbohydrate (lactose) and drinking too much at one time can raise your blood glucose levels. Curd or plain yogurt can be a better choice to meet your protein and calcium requirements without increasing your blood glucose levels.

Limit fruit portions

Fruit is healthy and must be eaten during pregnancy, but it is recommended not to exceed more than the number of portions advised by your dietitian. Most of them will prescribe not more than two portions of fruit spaced out between meals.

Remember to eat only one portion of fruit at a time. Choose slightly unripe fruits and eat it with the peel wherever possible. Ensure that you wash the fruit well. A portion of fruit is either a small-sized fruit (that fits your fist), half of a large piece of fruit, or about half a cup of fruit. Space out your fruits and have it in between meals as a mid-meal snack rather than immediately after the meal. Have a handful of almonds and walnuts with the fruit to give you satiety and maintain blood glucose levels.

Walnut consumption has also shown to curb cravings for unhealthy foods and improve insulin action

Real life example

Jyoti (name changed) was diagnosed with diabetes during her pregnancy. She was on two insulin shots a day. Jyoti was extra careful with her diet and never ate any outside food. She ate everything that was cooked at home using moderate oil and had fruits.

In spite of following a healthy meal plan, her blood glucose levels were always very high. During the conversation, she revealed that she ate 4–5 fruits each day assuming they were healthy. She had fruits whenever she was hungry, or had a craving for anything sweet. Additionally she added fruits to her salad to make them more nutritious.

Though fruits are healthy, portion control is important. They should ideally be taken as a snack and not combined with meals.

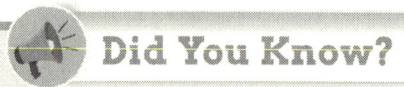

Fruit is preferred over fruit juice

It takes several fruits to make a glass of juice. As it is a concentrated source of carbohydrate in liquid form, it can raise blood glucose levels rapidly. A fruit instead has more fibre and also gives you a feeling of satiety keeping you full longer.

Strictly limit sweets, sweetened beverages, aerated drinks and desserts

Cakes, cookies, Indian sweets and pastries are a concentrated source of carbohydrate and fat that offer very little nutrition. It is best to avoid them. Do not add sugar, jaggery or honey to your foods as they are all a source of sugar and will result in high blood glucose levels.

Real life example

Sejal (name changed) is a Gujarati and had developed gestational diabetes in the 24th week of pregnancy. She came to me for nutrition planning as her blood glucose levels were not in the satisfactory range. During the conversation, she said their traditional food is cooked using sugar and is sweet. However the doctor had advised her against using sugar in any form direct or indirect so she had avoided it altogether. But a few moments later she confessed that she did not like the food that was cooked without sugar. Hence she was using the natural and healthy alternatives such as jaggery and honey. She added that these were organic products and she assured me that they were not the ones which are easily available in the market which has added sugar.

Here was the culprit that was disturbing her blood glucose levels. Though jaggery and honey were organic, they are a source of carbs and can increase the blood glucose levels. When I explained to her the effect of honey and jaggery on her blood glucose levels and how it would affect the health of the baby in turn, she was more than willing to change her diet to ensure good health of the baby.

> When a product says it is "sugar-free," take a closer look at the food label

It is advisable to check the food label on the product for the total carbohydrate and fat content before consuming it.

Limit intake of artificial sweeteners

Experts believe that using FDA approved artificial sweeteners is generally safe for women during pregnancy. Sucralose and Stevioside (stevia) are permitted to be used in moderate amounts. I suggest you consult your doctor or dietitian for more information.

Keep a food diary

Be sure to record all of the foods and the amount that you eat each day. This will help you monitor your carbohydrate intake. You can share this with your doctor and dietitian for review.

Real life example

Dhriti (name changed) was diagnosed with diabetes during her pregnancy and her HbA1c was also very high. Her doctor asked her to meet a dietitian and make the necessary changes in her meal plan to avoid complications in her pregnancy. Dhriti was a foodie by nature and she liked eating good food. She came to me for consultation during the festival season. She shared that she had a lot of craving for eating sweet food. She added that she had been cheating on her diet and had jalebis while taking an extra shot of insulin. However her blood glucose levels were still high.

I made her realize that taking the extra shot and eating food is not the right approach to eating foods that are restricted. As jalebi is made from refined flour, fried and then soaked in sugar syrup, there is a tendency that it raises blood glucose even after a few hours of consumption. So even though she was taking the extra shot her blood glucose levels would be high for a few hours.

Here are a few meal options which are recommended

Breakfast

- Egg (Boiled, poached, omelette, Spanish omelette with vegetables)
- Oats and Soya pancake/dosa
- Moong dal Chilla/Dosa/Pudla with Buttermilk/Curd
- Moong dal with vegetables paniyarams
- Broken wheat upma with vegetables and sprouts
- Moong dal idli/Oats idlis with coriander mint chutney/Yogurt chutney
- Egg Wrap/Paneer Wrap/vegetable wrap (use multigrain atta for the wrap)
- Vegetable dal paratha with curd

Lunch and Dinner

- Clear Unstrained Soups/Rasam and Stir fry vegetables
- Multigrain Roti/brown rice/Broken wheat (daliya)
- Green Vegetable
- Kadhi (dahi curry)/Dal/Whole Pulse (Sprouts, Ussal)/Fish/chicken (de-skinned)/Egg
- Curd/Buttermilk

Snacks

- Curd/Plain yogurt
- Boiled Egg
- Soya Nuts
- Roasted Chana with peanuts
- Chana Chaat/Sprouts with vegetables
- Makhana/Foxnuts, Jowar/bajra puffs, kurmura (rice puffs) with chana and vegetables
- Pulse based khakra (moong khakra, moth beans khakra)

It is important to meet a qualified dietitian to have your diet assessed. The dietitian will calculate the amount of carbohydrate, fat and protein that you need at meals and snacks and plan a customised meal plan for you.

Monitoring in GDM

The goal of management in gestational diabetes is to maintain blood glucose as near to normal as possible. Your doctor will ask you to regularly check your blood glucose levels using a blood glucose monitoring device.

You may also be recommended a continuous glucose monitoring (CGM)/Ambulatory glucose profile (AGP) test. CGMS/AGP is a device which records glucose readings once every 5–15 minutes and is usually inserted for a period of six days to 14 days. This will help your doctor and you understand how your blood glucose levels fluctuate throughout the day and night and make appropriate diet and medication changes if necessary.

Your monitoring program should include an HbA1c (glycosylated haemoglobin) test. This is a measure of your average blood glucose level over the past three months and is the gold standard for diabetes control. Your doctor will tell you when and how often you need to do this test.

In addition, to blood glucose testing, you may also be asked to check your urine for ketones. Ketones are by-products of the breakdown of fat and may be found in the blood and urine as a result of inadequate insulin or from inadequate calories in your diet.

What is self – blood glucose monitoring?

Once you are diagnosed as having gestational diabetes, your doctor will want to know more about your day-to-day blood glucose levels. As your pregnancy progresses, the placenta will release more of the hormones that work against insulin causing blood glucose spikes. Regular blood glucose monitoring is the key to giving you the information you need to effectively manage your diabetes.

Without regular testing, you will not know how well your diet, exercise, or medication are working. Blood glucose testing tells you and your doctor if you are on the right track or if you need to make changes. Testing your blood glucose level at important times during the day will help determine if proper diet and weight gain have kept blood glucose levels normal or if extra insulin is needed to help keep the baby protected.

The goals for blood glucose in gestational diabetes are usually stringent as it is important for a complication-free pregnancy and optimum growth and development of the baby.

The target blood glucose ranges are as follows

Fasting and pre-meal blood glucose < 90 mg/dL (5 mmol/l) and either

One hour post-meal < 140 mg/dL (7.8 mmol/l) or

Two-hour post-meal < 120 mg/dL (6.7 mmol/l)

HbA1c < 6% to be achieved without hypoglycaemia (low blood glucose)

How often and when should I test?

You may need to test your blood four to seven times a day. Generally, these times are fasting (first thing in the morning before you eat), before meals and one to two hours after the start of the meals. Occasionally, you may be asked to test more frequently during the day or at night.

Talk to your doctor/diabetes educator about setting appropriate target ranges and fitting a regular, well-defined blood glucose testing schedule for you.

Fasting tests

A fasting test can tell you if your insulin and bedtime snack are keeping you at safe blood glucose levels overnight. If your fasting glucose levels are high, the chances are that you may have had a low blood glucose level in the middle of the night. When on insulin, checking blood glucose at 3 A.M. is recommended.

Testing around meals

Measuring and controlling post-meal glucose is critical during pregnancy to avoid post-meal spikes. Testing before breakfast, lunch and dinner can help you decide on appropriate foods, portion sizes and dosage of your insulin or medication

Food is one of the main factors that directly impact your blood glucose levels and one that you can control. Checking blood glucose levels around mealtimes (before and one to two hours after a meal) gives you feedback on how your previous meal has affected your blood glucose levels. It helps you understand how your body reacts to specific foods and amounts, so that you can make informed choices about what to eat.

Real life example

Ketaki (name changed) had gestational diabetes and she was put on the insulin pump as her blood glucose levels were not manageable. She was putting in a lot of effort and would monitor her blood glucose levels frequently to understand the impact of food on her blood glucose levels.

She loved eating poha (rick flakes) but she found that whenever she ate poha, her blood glucose levels would go high after 3–4 hours. She came to me to understand if there was a way she could cook poha without her blood glucose levels going up. I gave her many options few of which being that she could eat a whole egg before eating the poha, or make dadpe pohe or curd pohe (dahi pohe) which was a better alternative to the regular poha.

Ketaki followed the instructions and sent me a message that implementing the given suggestions helped manage her blood glucose levels while she still enjoyed the poha.

Know your diet target

Diet target is the difference between your post-meal and pre-meal blood glucose. If the difference between the before and after meal readings is as per the diet target set for you, it indicates that the food choices and portions are working well. Please speak to your doctor/diabetes educator to know what should be the ideal difference for you.

Blood glucose monitors and CGMS/AGP are becoming more and more affordable, simple and easy to use. They give you a feedback in real-time where you, your dietitian and your doctor can make necessary changes to the diet or medication to ensure that your blood glucose levels are in range ensuring you have a safe and healthy pregnancy and delivery.

Pregnancy is a kind of "stress test" that often predicts future risk of diabetes. In one large study more than half of all women who had gestational diabetes developed Type 2 diabetes within 15 years of pregnancy. Because of the risk of developing Type 2 diabetes in the future, you should have your blood glucose level checked when you see your doctor for your routine check-ups. There is a good chance you will be able to reduce the risk of developing diabetes later in life by maintaining ideal body weight, eating healthy, exercising regularly, managing stress and sleeping well.

Real life journey shared by Hermeet Kaur

During my first pregnancy, I was diagnosed with gestational diabetes in the 26–27 weeks of pregnancy. When I conceived, my fasting blood glucose level was 101 mg/dl. My doctor had advised to control sugar intake. I took it as a general advice and did not understand the implications. My father has diabetes, so I always checked my glucose levels, but I had never seen even a borderline level in the earlier routine tests.

I had lots of cravings for spicy food as well as sweets. And I had in mind that a pregnant lady should eat whatever she enjoys as long it is hygienic. Because I never paid heed to the carbs or sugar intake, the levels probably shot up.

My fasting blood sugar went up to 121mg/dl, PP breakfast was 160–170 mg/dl. I was never told to get a glucose tolerance test done though. I always did fasting and PP 1 hour levels. I was referred to an endocrinologist who suggested a few dietary changes but that did not help, so I was put on insulin. 8 units per day-breakfast 2 units, lunch 4 units and dinner 2 units. This was increased to 20 units towards the end of my pregnancy. With insulin, I was able to keep the levels under 140 mg/dl in PP one hour tests. I would do three to four blood tests with a glucose monitor every day and report to the doctor.

Breakfast PP was always a challenge because no matter what I ate the level would always be closer to 150 mg/dl. With milk also the levels would increase. My daughter was 3 kgs at birth, healthy but she had difficulty maintaining the oxygen levels in blood and had mild

Respiratory Distress Syndrome. This was the side effect of me having gestational diabetes. She was kept in NICU for three days to stabilize. That time was super scary. If only I had known that my eating habits were of such importance, I would definitely be more careful. My blood glucose levels returned to normal immediately after the delivery. But I remained conscious of the sugar levels and consulted my dietitian who helped me keep my blood glucose levels and weight in check.

At the beginning of my second pregnancy, I immediately consulted my dietitian and she planned a diet and followed up regularly with me. My HbA1C level was maintained at 5.6%, fasting blood glucose well below 90 mg/dl and 1 hour post meals below 100 mg/dl. My doctor was very happy with my progress as I did not gain too much weight . I delivered a healthy baby boy without any complications. A healthy diet and regular physical activity can ensure a healthy pregnancy in GDM.

> **The principles of dietary management shared in this chapter can be followed by pregnant women with pre-existing diabetes (type 1 and type 2.)**

CHAPTER 12 Exercise

When it comes to diabetes, one of the misconceptions people with diabetes have is regarding exercise. For a lot of people, diabetes translates to an inability to exercise or a source of danger to the blood glucose levels. The truth couldn't be further away! In reality, exercise plays a huge role in supporting healthy blood glucose levels and enhancing the quality of life for a person living with diabetes

Exercise has a very important role to play in the management of diabetes. I always tell my patients that exercise itself works like insulin, helping maintain blood glucose levels in the optimum range. It helps to increase the good cholesterol (HDL) and reduces bad cholesterol (LDL) and blood pressure levels, thereby keeping the heart healthy and fit. It helps to preserve bone mass and builds and tones muscles. Exercise also increases your happy hormones making you feel better through the day and enhances your sense of wellbeing.

People with diabetes have high levels of glucose in their blood. Exercise or a form of physical activity helps the muscles use glucose without insulin. Thus, for people with Type 1 diabetes, whose beta cells are unable to produce insulin, exercise helps nourish the muscles with their glucose requirements adequately and keeps blood glucose levels in check. In addition, exercise can also help protect from lifestyle diseases and complications such as heart disease, kidney disease and other ailments which are a concern with a chronic condition such as diabetes.

Precautions before starting a workout regime

Consult your doctor before you start a new regimen. Your doctor may like to test for heart health, hypertension and other medical conditions before suggesting the suitable exercise forms for you. In addition, some people may be at risk for blocked or narrow arteries which may require close monitoring for certain exercises. Based on your medical history, your doctor, dietitian, diabetes educator and trained physical trainer will be able to suggest the ideal regimen for you.

In case you have been inactive, start slow! Most people get motivated and want to run a marathon on the first day itself, leading to further complications. Start small and give your body time to adjust to the new regimen. While pushing yourself is good, over-exertion all of a sudden can further wreak havoc on your blood glucose levels.

In addition, it is important to set realistic goals for yourself on a day-to-day basis. Again your doctor and diabetes educator can help you with this. Work on building your stamina and endurance over time instead of trying to get it all done instantly and getting demotivated.

Finally, an important thing to note before you start your new regimen is to keep access to some carbs, about 15 grams, in case you start feeling low. This will allow you to help stabilise your blood glucose in case of any sudden dips. Always carry your glucose monitor, ketone strips, glucose tablets or sugar to the gym or at your workout place to manage a hypoglycemic condition if it occurs. Also be sure to monitor your blood glucose levels closely before, during and after exercise to know the impact on your levels.

Be sure to drink enough water through the day as adequate hydration during exercise helps in maintaining fluid balance in the body.

If you are on insulin, you must ensure you have eaten a meal and are not exercising during the insulin peak time. Your doctor or diabetes educator will guide you on the peak time of insulin that you are taking.

You should not use the exercising part like thigh or arms for injecting insulin. Instead, another site such as abdomen or buttocks can be used to avoid the risk of hypoglycaemia.

Types of exercises

There is a wide range of exercises one can choose from to strengthen the body and be fit while also having some fun. These may be gentle exercises, aerobic exercises, HIIT (High-intensity interval training) exercises and strength training. Based on your condition, you can choose one or a combination of these for maximum benefits.

Gentle exercises such as yoga or pilates are easy on your muscles and joints while ensuring your body is stretched and worked out efficiently to strengthen muscles and boost blood circulation. Aerobic exercises include walking, jogging, zumba, swimming, cycling and similar others. On the other hand, HIIT exercises can be quite intensive and require a lot more energy and stamina while also boosting your metabolism. These include martial arts, cross-training and high-intensity sports like football.

American Diabetes Association recommends, aiming for 30 minutes of moderate-to-vigorous intensity aerobic exercise at least 5 days a week or a total of 150 minutes per week. The activity should be spread out over at least 3 days during the week and should not be skipped for more than 2 days together. Moderate intensity means that one is working hard enough that you can talk, but not sing, during the activity.

After getting used to a regular form of aerobic exercise in your daily regime, it is equally important to focus on strength training. This focuses on toning and strengthening your muscles and bones. This is especially important for people with diabetes as with muscles making more use of glucose, the levels in the blood tend to normalise. Weight training or push up using one's own body weight are great forms of strength training.

We Indians have low muscle mass and high-fat mass especially visceral fat, therefore making insulin action ineffective. To help insulin work better, it is important for us to work on improving muscle mass and reducing body fat stores especially abdominal fat. It is therefore recommended to do strength training at least 2 times per week in addition to aerobic activity. However it must be done only after a thorough screening and recommendation by your treating physician/diabetologist.

Below are examples of strength training activities that can be done without going to the gym:

- Using resistance bands
- Using one's own bodyweight like squats, lunges, push-ups, sit-ups, planks
- Lifting light weights or objects like canned goods or water bottles at home
- Other activities that build and keep muscle like cleaning the bathroom, mopping the house etc.

When it comes to setting up an exercise regime, it may be difficult at first but soon your body and overall health will start to respond positively. Pick a form you enjoy to help you stay motivated. You can even join a group class (though make sure you inform all the instructors about your condition) or even meet up with your friends for a walk. The important point to remember is not to get discouraged but stick with it long-term to reap maximum benefits.

Care tips when exercising

1. Exercise should always be initiated slowly and intensity should be increased gradually.
2. A warm-up period of stretching and other gentle activity and a final cool-down period must be followed.

Warm-up period: 5 to 10 minutes of aerobic activity such as walking, stretching or cycling at low intensity. The warm-up period is to prepare the muscles, heart and lungs for more intense activity that will follow.

Cool-down period: 5 to 10 minutes of aerobic activity such as walking, stretching or cycling at low intensity to be performed after a period of intense activity. The purpose is to gradually bring the heart rate down to the pre-exercise level.

3. Before starting any exercise program, you must have a thorough medical evaluation for the presence of macro and micro-vascular complications, so that your doctor and dietitian/diabetes educator can prescribe the best suited activity.

4. In the presence of proliferative or severe non-proliferative diabetic retinopathy, vigorous aerobic or resistance exercise may be contraindicated because of the potential risk of triggering vitreous haemorrhage or retinal detachment.

5. In the presence of severe peripheral neuropathy and diabetes kidney disease, it may be best to perform non-weight-bearing activities such as swimming, bicycling, or arm exercises.

6. You must ensure that you are well hydrated before, during and after exercise.

An imbalance in carbohydrate-protein intake and/or medication relative to exercise can result in disturbed blood glucose levels and muscle breakdown. When you experience low or high blood glucose levels pre, during or post-exercise, a record of activity and its intensity should be maintained. This helps your doctor, dietitian and diabetes educator to understand the need for a change in the medication and meal plan.

Hypoglycaemia (low blood glucose) can be a concern for people taking insulin or certain oral medications for diabetes which causes low blood glucose levels. Proper regulation of dosage of medication, amount and timings of meals and exercise should be planned with the help of your doctor and diabetes educator.

Dressing and footwear for the workout

- You must avoid tight-fitting outfits especially over hips or joints which can affect nerves resulting in pain or tingling during exercise.

- Exercising barefoot, with uncomfortable footwear or lack of smooth linings inside the shoe must be avoided.

- It is advisable to wear clean absorbent socks that do not have tight elastics at the top and are above the ankle.

- Always check your feet for injury before and after exercise especially in case of sores or blisters on the feet.

Self-Monitoring of Blood Glucose (SMBG) and exercise

Doing SMBG (Self-Monitoring Blood Glucose) before, during and after exercise helps to understand the effect of medication, diet and exercise on the blood glucose levels.

It is best to avoid exercise if:

- Blood glucose level is > 240 mg/dl (13.3 mmol/l)

- Blood glucose level is < 70 mg/dl (3.9 mmol/l) (hypoglycaemia)

- In type 1 diabetes, if fasting blood glucose level is > 250 mg/dl (13.9 mmol/l) and/or ketones are positive.

- If your blood glucose level is below 100 mg/dl (5.6 mmol/l) before exercise you must eat and go. Delay exercise till blood glucose levels reach upto 90–100 mg/dl (5–5.6 mmol/l)

- When blood glucose levels are below 100–120 mg/dl (5.6–6.7 mmol/l), you can consume a 10–20 g carbohydrate snack like an egg/paneer wrap or a fruit (banana/mango will do) with nuts or oats porridge before exercising.

It is advisable to do self-monitoring of blood glucose after every 30 minutes of high-intensity exercise, as blood glucose levels may rise due to an increase in stress hormones. In such cases, it is also important to check for ketones in the urine and accordingly stop the exercise immediately.

During the initial days of starting an exercise, you should check the blood glucose levels during the workout to rule out hypoglycaemia.

If your blood glucose levels fall below 80mg/dl (4.4 mmol/l), you should have glucose tablets or sugar to correct hypoglycaemia immediately and care should be taken to modify the pre-workout snack or medication or timing of exercise to avoid these episodes in the future.

Never check the blood glucose levels immediately post-exercise. There are high chances that the blood glucose monitor will show a high reading as the body is under stress during and immediately post-workout. Allow the body to cool down before you check blood glucose levels.

A continuous glucose monitoring system/ambulatory glucose profile is the best bet when embarking on a new exercise regime as it gives you a complete picture of how your blood glucose is responding to exercise not only during but also later. This will help make the necessary tweaks in medication, diet etc. and avoid hypo/hyperglycaemia episodes.

Exercise is the cornerstone in diabetes management and must be done by everyone. We have even our patients with type 1 diabetes who are on multiple insulin regimes or insulin pump therapy run ultra-marathons, triathlons, treks etc. DO NOT LET DIABETES STOP YOU FROM

EXERCISING. Take out one hour from your 24 hour day to indulge in a physical activity of your choice. Make sure your "Me time" is fun. Begin today and reap its health benefits and enjoy a great sense of wellbeing.

Real life example

Parul (name changed) has been dealing with Type 1 diabetes for many years and at 32 years of age, her weight was 70kgs. While I have been counselling her on her diet for a few months now, I realised she has quite a sedentary lifestyle and does not participate in any exercise or physical activity. When I asked her about it, she said she was scared as she is too weak or worries that her workout may drastically impact her blood glucose levels.

I then checked her random blood glucose level which was at 220 mg/dl (12.2 mmol/l) and advised her to first get her blood glucose levels in range by correcting her insulin dosage and meal plan.

I then suggested that she must start walking at a medium pace for 15 minutes a day and after a week to build it up to 20 minutes a day. She was advised to include a suitable warm-up and cool-down routine each time to avoid any injury or sudden spikes in her blood glucose levels. I also advised her to keep a log of her blood glucose levels before, during and after her workouts.

After a few weeks when her confidence and stamina improved, she started walking at a brisk pace for 30 minutes a day. When she came back to me, next she was very happy as her weight had reduced by 4 kg. She was active and energetic and found that her blood glucose levels were stabilising.

CHAPTER 13   Get Label Wise

Nutrition management is very important to maintain optimum blood glucose levels. Avoiding fried food, counting calories, counting carbohydrates, planning meal times – all these seem to be trending today. In many cases, people with diabetes go a step further by spending hours at grocery aisles trying to make sense of food labels and picking up healthy packets. Regular chips and soda cans are replaced with diet-friendly foods, and traditional home-cooked meals with 'diabetes friendly' meal options. Yet frustratingly, many a times these changes just don't seem to reflect on the blood glucose levels.

This is where a lack of understanding of the food labels comes in. Picking up boxes which have words like 'sugar-free', 'diet', 'baked not fried' and even 'diabetes friendly' may seem like the healthier options, but seldom are in reality. Taking a deeper look at the food label and understanding the actual composition of the ingredients like sugar, refined flour or fat per serving can help you make a better choice

When you go grocery shopping, if you check just about every packaged food available today has a food label indicating the serving size and other nutritional information. The "nutrition facts" food labels are intended to give you information about the specific packaged food in question. Measurements of fat, cholesterol, sodium, carbohydrate, protein, vitamins, and minerals are calculated for a "typical portion size". It is recommended that every time you are at a grocery store, you take that extra minute to look at the food labels of the items you are buying. Reading the label is the only way to know what you are eating.

A few tips on how to read Food labels

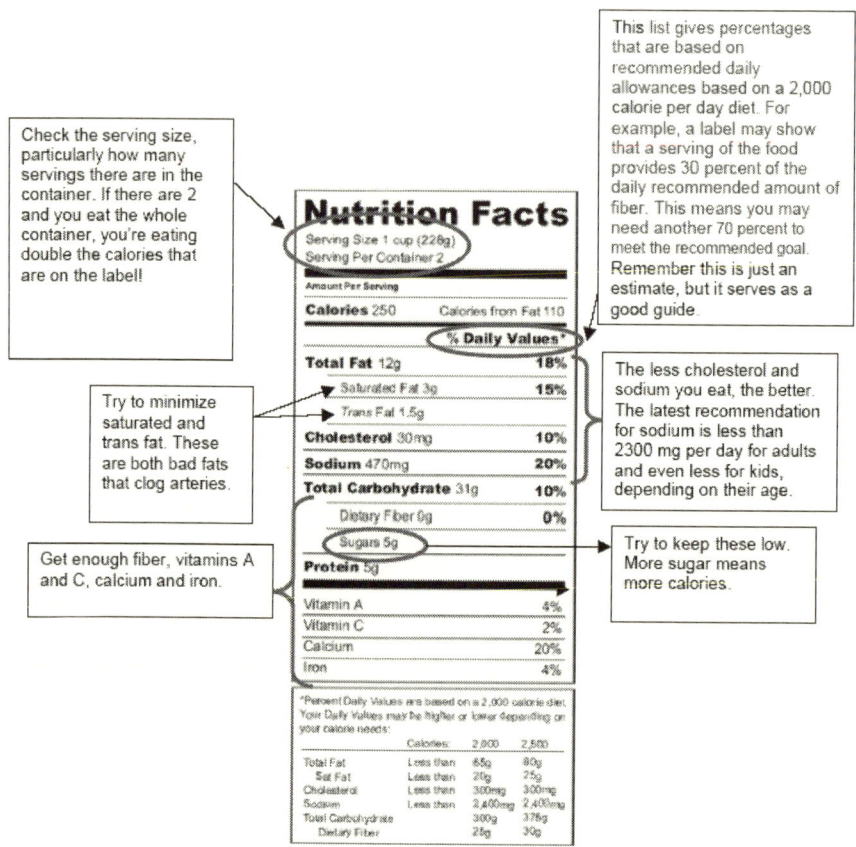

On May 20, 2016, the FDA announced the new nutrition facts label for packaged foods to reflect new scientific information, including the link between diet and chronic diseases such as obesity and heart disease.

Get Label Wise

Nutrition Facts (Original label)

Serving Size 2/3 cup (55g)
Servings Per Container About 8

Amount Per Serving

Calories 230	Calories from Fat 72

	% Daily Value*
Total Fat 8g	12%
Saturated Fat 1g	5%
Trans Fat 0g	
Cholesterol 0mg	0%
Sodium 160mg	7%
Total Carbohydrate 37g	12%
Dietary Fiber 4g	16%
Sugars 1g	
Protein 3g	
Vitamin A	10%
Vitamin C	8%
Calcium	20%
Iron	45%

* Percent Daily Values are based on a 2,000 calorie diet. Your daily value may be higher or lower depending on your calorie needs.

	Calories:	2,000	2,500
Total Fat	Less than	65g	80g
Sat Fat	Less than	20g	25g
Cholesterol	Less than	300mg	300mg
Sodium	Less than	2,400mg	2,400mg
Total Carbohydrate		300g	375g
Dietary Fiber		25g	30g

Nutrition Facts (New label)

8 servings per container
Serving size 2/3 cup (55g)

Amount per serving
Calories 230

	% Daily Value*
Total Fat 8g	10%
Saturated Fat 1g	5%
Trans Fat 0g	
Cholesterol 0mg	0%
Sodium 160mg	7%
Total Carbohydrate 37g	13%
Dietary Fiber 4g	14%
Total Sugars 12g	
Includes 10g Added Sugars	20%
Protein 3g	
Vitamin D 2mcg	10%
Calcium 260mg	20%
Iron 8mg	45%
Potassium 235mg	6%

* The % Daily Value (DV) tells you how much a nutrient in a serving of food contributes to a daily diet. 2,000 calories a day is used for general nutrition advice.

Original label   **New label**

Ref: https://www.fda.gov/Food/GuidanceRegulation/GuidanceDocumentsRegulatoryInformation/LabelingNutrition/ucm385663.htm

Below are some explanations of its components.

1. **Serving size**

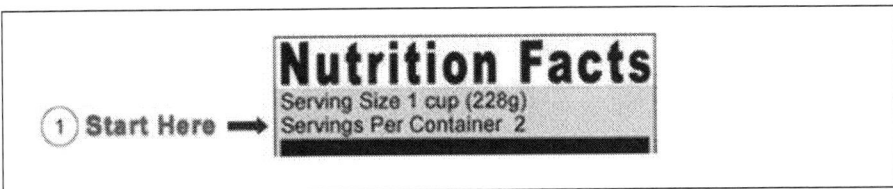

Ref:https://www.fda.gov/Food/IngredientsPackagingLabeling/LabelingNutrition/ucm274593.htm

Serving sizes are based on the amount of food people typically eat, which makes them realistic and easy to compare to similar foods. It is important to pay attention to the serving size, especially the number of servings in the package and that needs to be compared with the amount an individual actually eats out of the package. The size of the serving on the food package influences all the nutrient amounts listed on the top part of the label.

For example, if a package has 4 servings and one eats half the package, which is 2 servings, it means the individual has consumed double the calories, fats, and other nutrients mentioned on the label (amount per serving)

Real life example

Neha (name changed) was obese and had type 2 diabetes. She had been asked by her doctor to lose weight to bring down her blood glucose levels. In an attempt to jumpstart her weight loss regime and eat healthy, she decided to eat one meal that consisted of ready-to-eat cereal every day. The box claimed to promote weight loss and offer daily nutrition as well. Yet after a month or so of following the new diet, she had not lost any weight, nor had her blood glucose levels dropped.

Disheartened, she came to me for consultation. While she was sharing her meal plan she shared, "I have been on a diet for an entire month hence gave up on eating my regular food and ate cereals for my main meals as well. I eat home-cooked food only for lunch and still my body is not supporting me. I am not able to lose any weight nor is my blood glucose coming under control. I am feeling demotivated as all the efforts I am putting in are giving no results."

On listening to her story I knew where she was going wrong. I explained the food label to her and made her understand that the amount of sugar and refined flour in the cereal she was consuming was way more than she should be eating. Further, as the proportions were given per serving size (which was much smaller than what Neha was used to eating) she was consuming almost double the calories she initially assumed.

At this point, I made changes to her meal plan, incorporated food items she liked to eat and explained the proportions and type of the cereal that she should be eating. She looked at me with doubt in her eyes. I asked her to follow this plan and check her weight and blood glucose levels after a fortnight.

A couple of weeks later, she sent me a message that she had lost 1 ½ kg and her blood glucose levels were showing a normal trend.

2. **Calories (and Calories from Fat)**

Calories provide a measure of how much energy and nutrients you get for the stated serving size. This is the part of the food label where you will find the amount of fat per serving. The number of servings you consume determines the number of calories you actually eat (your portion amount).

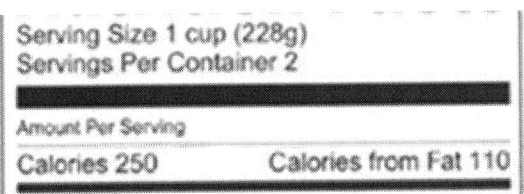

For example, if there are 250 calories in one serving of spaghetti with cheese, 110 calories come from fat which means almost half the calories in a single serving, came from fat.

What if you ate the whole package content? Then, you would consume two servings, or 500 calories and 220 calories would come from fat.

General Guide to Calories

- 40 Calories are low
- 100 Calories are moderate
- 400 Calories or more are high

The General Guide to Calories provides a general reference for calories when you look at a nutrition facts label. This guide is based on a 2,000 calorie diet.

3. **The Nutrients: How much?:** This section shows some key nutrients that impact health and separates them into two main groups:
   - Limit These Nutrients
   - Get Enough of These

Limit These Nutrients

- Total fat
- Saturated fat
- Trans-fat
- Cholesterol
- Sodium

Limit these Nutrients	
Total Fat 12g	**18%**
Saturated Fat 3g	15%
Trans Fat 3g	
Cholesterol 30mg	**10%**
Sodium 470mg	**20%**

Ref:https://www.fda.gov/Food/IngredientsPackagingLabeling/LabelingNutrition/ucm274593.htm

It is recommended to keep the intake of saturated fat, trans-fat, cholesterol, sodium and simple sugars to as low as possible as part of a nutritionally balanced diet.

Guidelines to tell if food is high in fat, saturated fat, salt or sugar

	Sugar	Total Fat	Saturated fat	Salt
	(Per 100 g of product)			
High	More than 22.5 g	More than 17.5 g	More than 5 g	More than 1.5 g (or 0.6 g sodium)
Medium	Between 5 g and 22.5 g	Between 3 g and 17.5 g	Between 5 g and 1.5 g	Between 0.3 and 1.5 g
Low	5 g and less	3 g and less	1.5 g and less	0.3 g and less (or 0.1 g sodium)

Ref:https://www.fssai.gov.in/dam/jcr:4a9bc826.../Note_Report_HFSS_08_05_2017.pdf

Get Enough of These

a. Dietary fibre

b. Vitamin A

c. Vitamin C

d. Calcium

e. Iron

Get Enough of These	
Dietary Fiber 0g	0%
Vitamin A	4%
Vitamin C	2%
Calcium	20%
Iron	4%

Ref:https://www.fda.gov/Food/IngredientsPackagingLabeling/LabelingNutrition/ucm274593.htm

Most of us do not get enough dietary fibre, vitamin A, vitamin C, calcium, and iron in our diets. Eating enough of these nutrients can improve your health and help reduce the risk of some diseases and conditions. For example, getting enough calcium may reduce the risk of osteoporosis, a condition that results in brittle bones as one ages. Eating a diet high in dietary fibre promotes healthy bowel function and reduces cholesterol and weight and improves blood glucose levels.

4. **Carbohydrate Count**

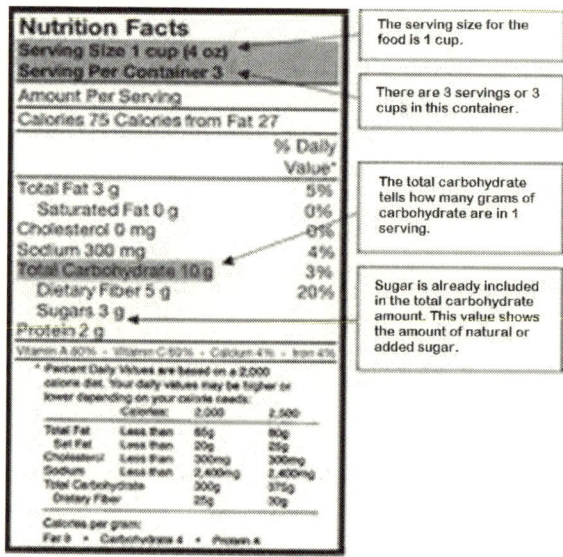

Total carbohydrates

For individuals with diabetes, it is most important to be able to use the information given regarding carbohydrate on the label in the most appropriate way. Total carbohydrate, is the amount of carbohydrate present per serving of the food. If you eat two servings, you can multiply the total carbohydrate per serving into two.

Total carbohydrate on the label includes all types of carbohydrate – sugar (both natural and added), complex carbohydrate and fibre.

Beneath the Total Carbohydrates line, there will be two or three other lines – fibre, sugars, and sometimes sugar alcohols.

Sugar

Sugar is included in the total carbohydrate amount. A check has to be kept on the amount of carbohydrates coming from sugar. This number must be as low as possible. Different brands and products can be compared and the ones with the lowest number of sugar grams per serving must be chosen. According to the latest amendments suggested by the FDA, "Added Sugars" will also be included under "Total Sugars" to help consumers understand how much sugar has been added to the product. To keep the sugar intake minimum, care has to be taken that added sugars are not listed as one of the first few ingredients. Other names for added sugars include: corn syrup, high-fructose corn syrup, fruit juice concentrate, maltose, dextrose, sucrose, jaggery, honey, and maple syrup.

Artificial (Non-Nutritive) sweeteners are high-intensity sweeteners providing negligible nutrients and calories and are approved by the Food and Drug Administration (FDA) for use.

Examples of artificial sweeteners are acesulfame K, aspartame, neotame, saccharin, sucralose and stevioside (stevia).

Saccharin is not recommended for use in pregnant women and children. It is not heat stable.

Aspartame is not recommended for use in children, children with phenylketonuria and is restricted in pregnant women with hyperphenylalaninemia. It is not heat stable.

Acesulfame potassium must be used with caution in individuals on potassium restricted diet (kidney disease) or having sulfa antibiotic based allergy. It is heat stable.

Sucralose and Stevioside (stevia) have no specific side effects and are considered to be safe for consumption in children as well as pregnant women. They are both heat stable and can be used in cooking.

Check with your dietitian/doctor on the amount of sweetener permitted on a daily basis.

Sugar Alcohols

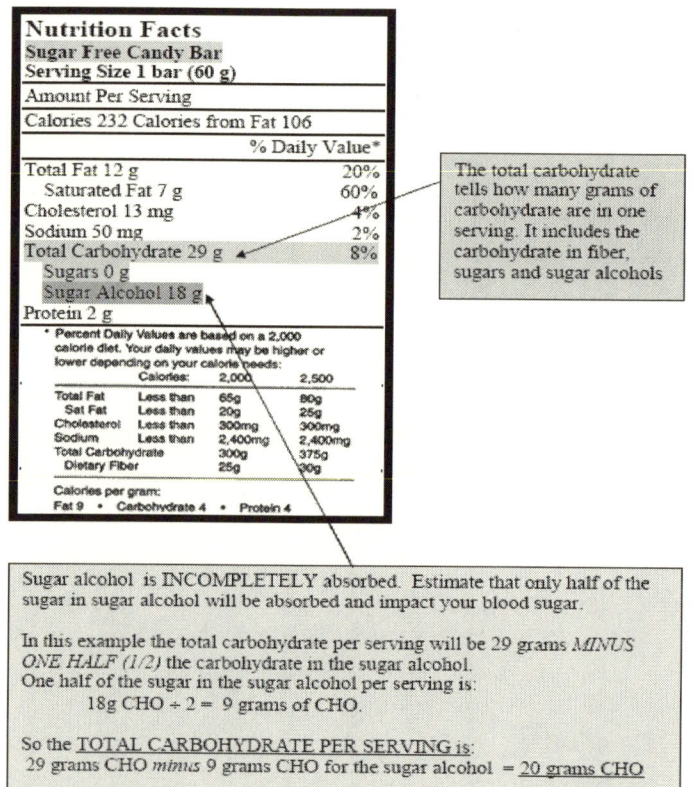

Ref:https://dtc.ucsf.edu/living-with-diabetes/diet-and-nutrition/understanding-carbohydrates/counting-carbohydrates/learning-to-read-labels/counting-sugar-alcohols/

Sugar alcohols are like sugar in some ways, but they are not completely absorbed by the body. Because of this, the impact of sugar alcohols on blood glucose levels is less and they provide fewer calories per gram. Names of the individual sugar alcohols will be present on the ingredient list of any product that contains them. They will be included in the amount of carbohydrate on the label, either in the total or on a separate line for sugar alcohols. If the product is labelled "sugar-free" or "no added sugar," the manufacturer must show the sugar alcohol count separately.

Note especially that many of the sugar alcohols aren't as sweet as sugar, so more may be used to get the same sweetness. Also, many sugar alcohols can cause gas and other adverse intestinal reactions because they are not completely digested.

Fibre

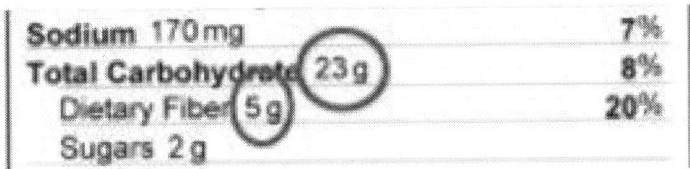

Fibre being indigestible carbohydrate does not raise blood glucose. In fact, the presence of fibre can slow down the impact of the other carbohydrates in a meal. Therefore, when counting carbs, subtract the fibre grams from the total grams of carbohydrate to get a more accurate estimate of the carbohydrate impact on the diet.

Total Carbohydrate (g)/serving − Fibre (g)/serving = Net Carbohydrates/serving

This gives a number which is called effective carbs, or usable carbs, or net carbs, or impact carbs.

For example, if a cereal has 23 grams of carbohydrate per serving, but also 5 grams of fibre. One can consider it to be only 18 grams of carbohydrate.

In some countries, they do not subtract the fibre from total carbohydrate. Check with your dietitian for more details.

5. **Ingredients**

Every food product will have a list of ingredients on the label. They are listed from largest to smallest amount (by weight). This means a food contains the largest amount of the first ingredient and the smallest amount of the last ingredient. It should also have a mention of the presence of common allergens like soy, peanuts, wheat (gluten) and milk (lactose).

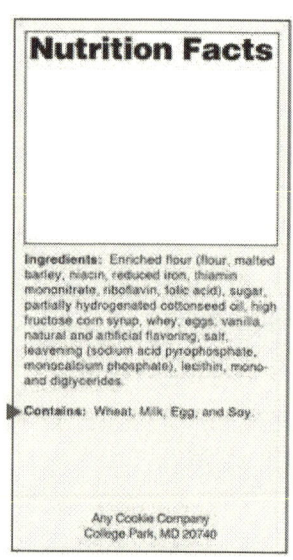

6. **Understanding Daily Value (DV)**

The % Daily Value (DV) tells the percentage of each nutrient in a single serving, in terms of the daily recommended amount. The daily recommended amounts may be provided as a footnote at the bottom of the label for a 2000 or 2500 calorie diet. Percent daily values are based on a 2000 calorie diet. For diets other than 2,000 calories, dividing by 2,000 helps to determine the % Daily Value for nutrients. For example, for a 1,500 calorie diet, the % Daily Value goal will be based on 75% for each nutrient, not 100%.

To consume less of a nutrient (such as saturated fat or sodium), one should choose a product with a lower % DV — 5 percent or less. To consume more of a nutrient (such as fibre), foods with a higher% DV — 20 percent or more should be chosen.

	% Daily Value*
Total Fat 12g	18%
Saturated Fat 3g	15%
Trans Fat 3g	
Cholesterol 30mg	10%
Sodium 470mg	20%
Total Carbohydrate 31g	10%
Dietary Fiber 0g	0%
Sugars 5g	
Protein 5g	
Vitamin A	4%
Vitamin C	2%
Calcium	20%
Iron	4%

Ref:https://www.fda.gov/Food/IngredientsPackagingLabeling/LabelingNutrition/ucm274593.htm

7. **Health Claims**

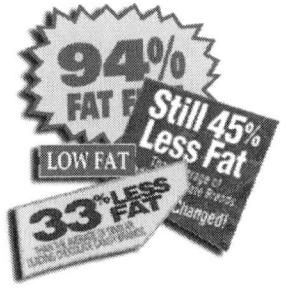

Some food labels make claims such as "low cholesterol" or "low fat." These claims can only be used if they meet the following criteria:

Guide for Label Claims

COMPONENT	CLAIM	NOT MORE THAN
Energy	Low	40 kcal (170 kJ) per 100 g (solids) Or 20 kcal (80 kJ) per 100 ml (liquids)
	Free	4 kcal per 100 ml (liquids)
Fat	Low	3 g per 100 g (solids) 1.5 g per 100 ml (liquids)
	Free	0.5 g per 100 g (solids) or 100 ml (liquids)
Saturated Fat	Low	1.5 g per 100 g (solids) 0.75 g per 100 ml (liquids) and 10% of energy
	Free	0.1 g per 100 g (solids) 0.1 g per 100 ml (liquids)
Cholesterol	Low	0.02 g per 100 g (solids) 0.01 g per 100 ml (liquids)
	Free	0.005 g per 100 g (solids) 0.005 g per 100 ml (solids) and, for both claims, less than: 1.5 g saturated fat per 100 g (solids) 0.75 g saturated fat per 100 ml (liquids) and 10% of the energy of saturated fat
Sugars	Low	5 g per 100 g (solids) 2.5 g per 100 ml (liquids)
	Free	0.5 g per 100 g (solids) 0.5 g per 100 ml (liquids)
Sodium	Low	0.12 g per 100 g
	Very Low	0.04 g per 100 g
	Free	0.005 g per 100 g

		NOT LESS THAN
Protein	Source	10% of NRV per 100 g (solids)
		5% of NRV per 100 ml (liquids)
		or 5% of NRV per 100 kcal (12% of NRV* per 1 MJ)
		or 10% of NRV per serving
	High	2 times the values for "source"
Vitamins and Minerals	Source	15% of NRV per 100 g (solids)
		7.5% of NRV per 100 ml (liquids)
		or 5% of NRV per 100 kcal (12% of NRV per 1 MJ)
		or 15% of NRV per serving
	High	2 times the value for "source"

*NRV-Nutrient Reference Value
Ref: CAC/GL 23–1997
http://www.fao.org/docrep/005/Y2770E/y2770e07.htm

Real life example

Priya (name changed) is a working woman and has type 2 diabetes for 4 years. Her blood glucose levels were erratic. Her doctor asked her to choose healthy options. As she worked late hours at the office, she decided to start carrying sandwiches made from 7-grain bread with her every day to avoid eating in the canteen. Even though she thought she was choosing a healthy food option, her pre-dinner blood glucose readings would always be high.

Priya came to my clinic to understand why her blood glucose readings were going high even after a vegetable sandwich made from healthy 7-grain bread. When I checked the food label of the bread, I was astonished to see that even though the label claimed to be a 7-grain bread, it had 70% refined flour (maida) and only 5% oats, 3% ragi and such, offering negligible quantities of the healthy ingredients. The high content of refined flour was instead causing her blood glucose levels to be quite high.

I advised Priya to switch to actual healthy and filling options such as dry bhel, boiled eggs, chana chaat (brown grams) and paneer tikka without extra butter for her evening snacks and then monitor her blood glucose levels.

After 10 days of following the new meal plan, she came back to me happy as with the same medications that she was taking, her blood glucose levels were in the normal range.

Hence, it is very important to read food labels when you eat packaged food.

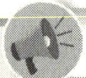 **Frequently Asked Question**

Busting the Myth – Brown Sugar is better than White Sugar

I have often seen people swap white sugar with brown sugar, assuming that it is a healthier option.

Let's understand the facts

Brown sugar is nothing but ordinary table sugar that is turned brown by the reintroduction of 5–10 percent molasses to improve the colour and taste. This usually appeals to people aesthetically, since it gives the "organic" appearance. Brown sugar has slightly more minerals than white sugar but not sufficient enough to reap any health benefits.

The carb and calorie content of both brown sugar and white sugar are the same

Real life example

Smriti (name changed), a homemaker, had been struggling with high blood glucose levels for a while now. When Smriti came to me for consultation, she revealed "I feel hungry even after eating my meals. My doctor has asked me to eat 6 small meals a day. I eat home-cooked food for my main meals viz. Breakfast, Lunch and Dinner, but for my mid-meal, I snack on diet foods that are available in the market (like diet chips, chivda, chakli and other snacks.)"

When I explained to her about food labels and discussed the nutrition content of the diet food she was eating, she was shocked to know that her diet foods were responsible for her high blood glucose levels. All diet foods have excess salt or sugar to enhance their flavour. So, in Smriti's case while the fat content may be slightly low, the sugar content was almost double that of what she should be having. Similarly, biscuits (oats/ragi/multigrain) that claim to be diabetes friendly and sugar-free are generally loaded with high amounts of fat to make up for the low sugar taste. This fat is quite harmful to health as it can raise LDL cholesterol levels (bad fat) in the body.

Thus, even though Smriti was trying to choose healthy options, all her processed packets were actually harming her diabetes treatment. I advised her to snack on roasted makhanas (fox nut/lotus seeds), jowar puffs, boiled egg or cucumber sticks with a dip which are healthy mid-meal snacks and do not raise blood glucose levels.

We often hear people say this "I am on a weight loss diet. I should stock up on 'Diet Foods'."

We see an entire section dedicated to these diet foods on the shelves of supermarkets and we mindlessly head straight to that section picking up stuff for our guilt-free snacking. Be aware of the fact that not all diet/health foods are genuine.

Those of us watching our waistlines choose brown bread over white bread thinking we are making a smart eating choice.

Beware! The truth is that the so-called brown bread may not necessarily be made with whole wheat flour or whole grain. Some manufacturers add caramel colour to the dough to give the brown colour to the bread. The soft texture of the brown bread is maintained by adding $3/4^{th}$ refined flour (maida) to $1/4^{th}$ wheat flour, so it is actually white bread in disguise which is even worse than the labelled white bread.

This holds true for the multigrain biscuits as well which may be low in sugar content but contain a large amount of unhealthy fat, without which they cannot be made crispy and crunchy. These fats can increase the risk of diabetes, heart disease and sudden cardiac death.

Now coming to our very popular roasted/diet snacks. Roasted does not mean its calorie or carbohydrate-free. Usually diet snacks available commercially are also higher in their sodium content to make it more palatable. To make matters worse, most of us end up finishing almost the entire packet of diet snacks sitting in front of the television assuming it is a healthier option.

There are two options available "low-fat" or "fat-free". The low-fat version is the one which is deep-fried but the oil is drained out. Fat-free is where they use refined edible oil to spray seasonings and enhance flavour. One quick exercise you could do is crushing some in a blotting paper and see if it stains with oil. Avoid these diet snacks which can jeopardize both your health and wealth as they are prized high.

Make sure you read the food labels to understand if they are really healthy or is it just another marketing gimmick.

8. **Food Product Dating**

The three most common dates are sell-by date, Use-By Date, and Expiration Date. But what do they mean?

Sell-By Date/Display until: Refers to the last day a retailer can display a product for sale. You should buy the product before the sell-by date expires. But you can still store it at home if refrigerated properly for some time beyond that date depending on the product.

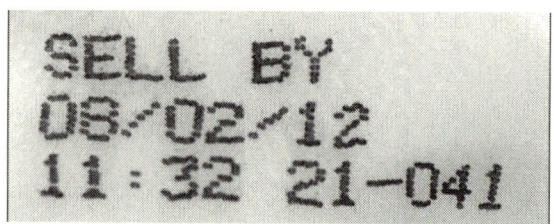

Use-By, Best if Used By, Best By, Best Before: Refers to the last day a product will maintain its optimum freshness, flavour, and texture. After the "use-by" or "best" date has passed, you may start to notice gradual changes in the unopened product's texture, colour, or flavour. But as long as the unopened item is handled properly and stored at 40 °F or below, it is generally considered safe to consume. This means, even if the date expires during home storage, a product should be wholesome, of good quality and safe to consume beyond this date. Your best bet for gauging whether an unopened shelf-stable product with this type of date is still of satisfactory quality is to simply smell and examine it first. Always discard foods that have developed an off odour, flavour or appearance.

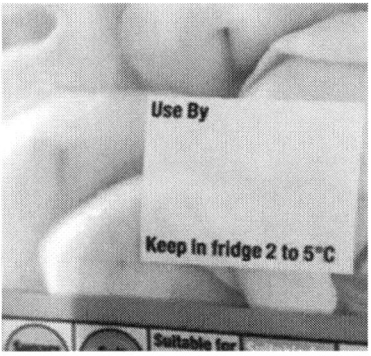

Expiration Date: You should always use the product before this date has passed. What this means is – if you haven't used a product by this date, discard it.

Packing codes: These codes, which appear as a series of letters and/or numbers on the package, sometimes indicate the date of manufacture. Packing codes help manufacturers and grocers rotate their stock and quickly locate products in the event of a recall.

Storage Tips

Here are a few tips on how to store the food and use it at top quality:

- Purchase the product before the sell-by date expires.
- Follow handling recommendations on product.
- If perishable, take the food home immediately after purchase and refrigerate it promptly. Freeze it if you can't use it within times recommended on the chart.
- Once a perishable product is frozen, it doesn't matter if the date expires because foods kept frozen continuously are safe indefinitely.

Research suggests that good use of nutrition labels is related to better nutrition knowledge, practice, and that overall use is linked to health motivation. Overall, nutrition labelling empowers you and allows for more healthful food choices.

CHAPTER 14
Eating out Options

Eating out is very common in today's modern life and for some, a way of life. As we spend most of our waking hours at work, we often end up eating out due to work commitments and business engagements. Dining out, weekend parties, ordering in, celebrating special occasions like birthdays, anniversaries, festivals, or a promotion – all call for outside food.

With each of these 'special occasions' becoming more and more common, our waistlines are increasing and health conditions worsening. Does this mean we stop eating out completely and restrict ourselves to 'diet homemade food?' The answer is `No'. Follow a simple thumb rule – keep it to once or twice a week, make wise choices and be watchful of how much you eat.

With technological advancements these days, menus and restaurant details are easily available online. Use this to your advantage by deciding what you are going to eat before you reach the venue. Avoid stepping out for dinner on an empty stomach as you may end up ordering more than you can eat. Instead, ensure you have a salad or a soup at home before you leave. Also, not all restaurant food is unhealthy. There are many items on the menu which can be cooked nutritiously and would not do much harm to your waistline or blood glucose levels. Call for the chef and give clear instructions of keeping the fat, sauces, salt and sugar to the minimum. He will be more than happy to oblige by suggesting healthy options and serving you a healthy meal.

When at a restaurant, keep these simple tips in mind that will help you dine out wisely without derailing your efforts to lose weight or be healthy.

- Eat portions similar to what you would eat at home
- Opt for steamed salads with lemon/mustard or vinegar dressings
- Request the chef to hold the cream, which is often put as a garnish over most soups. Avoid adding fried croutons to the soup
- Ask for smaller or half portions
- Skip appetisers, bread, and butter
- Skip the fries and mashed potatoes and order extra vegetables (e.g. sautéed spinach, grilled vegetables and mushrooms) on the side
- Ask for less sauce to be added to your meals. Sauces can be served on the side
- Request the chef not to add any cream, tadka of ghee or butter before serving
- Go low on salt as the extra salt in food could leave you feeling bloated
- Opt for ala carte instead of the buffet

Choose This	Skip This
Grilled, Poached, Boiled,	Fried-Deep fry or shallow fry
Steamed, Baked, Barbequed	Crispy, tempura, crunchy

Roasted, Lightly Stir-fried, Sautéed	Buttered, butter-fried, golden fried
Tandoori/Tikka	Batter Fried, tadka
Clear/Broth/Minestrone/Miso	Creamy/Cream of
Broiled	Cheesy
Red Sauce, Pesto Sauce	White Sauce, Pink Sauce
Vegetables sticks/Salad	Breadsticks, Fried Noodles, Croutons
Balsamic Vinegar, apple cider vinegar, lemon, Vinaigrette, hung curd, chilli vinegar, mustard dressing, salsa, guacamole and hummus	Ranch, Mayonnaise, Caesar, Blue Cheese, Sweet Onion, Italian, Cream dressing, Fondue, Tex-Mex dip, cheese dip
Jacket potato/grilled vegetables/Sautéed mushrooms, baked sweet potato	Mashed potato/French fries
Greek salad, Somtum (green papaya salad), fresh greens in vinaigrette/tossed in olive oil.	Caesar Salad, salads with Mayo dressing or high-fat sugar dressings
Buttermilk, salted lassi, mojito without sugar, lemon water(salted), coconut water, plain yogurt, curd	Freakshakes, milkshakes, cocktails, mocktails, aerated drinks, flavoured drinks and yogurts

Real life example

Neeti (name changed) is a 39-year-old lady with type 2 diabetes who enjoys a good social life like most young adults. She loves trying out new menus and spending time with friends. Having a great fondness for Punjabi food, she usually lands up at an Indian restaurant for a meal out and typically orders a naan along with dal makhani. While this sounds like a common choice for most people, Neeti found that her post-meal blood glucose levels would be extremely high and stay that way for a very long time. She was very particular about maintaining her blood glucose levels in the normal range and monitored them regularly. She came to me to understand how she could balance eating out without derailing her blood glucose levels.

After understanding her eating pattern and food choices she made when eating out, I told her that the maida content from the naan and high butter and fat content from the dal makhani were causing her blood glucose levels to spike dangerously and stay high for a long time.

I offered her options to choose while eating out. She was asked to opt for tandoori paneer or grilled chicken for starters, tandoori roti, missi roti or phulka without butter instead of the naan, choose lasuni palak instead of paneer makhanwala along with dal and a vegetable raita.

While eating out, the trick is to identify the right food options from the menu that will not affect your blood glucose levels drastically. Many a times, people choose certain dishes thinking they are a healthy option, but when they check their post-meal readings, they are extremely high. Knowing what to choose and what to avoid can allow you to enjoy a good social life without affecting your glucose levels.

Here are a few healthy options to choose from across various cuisines:

Healthy Options – Indian Cuisine

- Idli, Dal paniyaram, Pesarattu (moong dal) dosa with Sambar/Rasam
- Dhokla/Khandvi/Patra (less coconut and tadka)
- Tomato Omelette (Besan Omelette, Besan Chilla, Besan Pudla)
- Chana Chaat
- Chapati, Phulka, Tandoori Roti without butter, Missi Roti

- Plain Steamed Rice, Palak Khichdi, Dal Khichdi

- Rasam, Tomato Shorba, Sambar, Yellow Dal, Moong Dal, Panchratni Dal

- Chole, Methi Palak, Khumb (mushroom) Palak, Khumb Makai, Khumb Matar, Gobi Matar, Sabj Punch Mahal, Tandoori Gobi, Tawa Sabzi (Cooked in Less Oil)

- Chicken Tikka, Reshmi Kabab, Fish Tikka, Tangdi Kabab, Tandoori Chicken, Tawa Machli and Tawa Chicken

- Garden Salad, Leafy Sprout Salad, Tossed Mushrooms and Bell Peppers, Grilled/Sautéed Vegetable in Garlic

- Paneer Shaslik, Grilled Mix Vegetables, Spicy Paneer

- Palak Paneer (No Cream), Grilled Paneer Tikka

- Rajma/Chana Masala, Palak Lasuni, Veg Kolhapuri/Hyderabadi (Cooked in Less Oil)

> Request the chef not to baste the tandoori item with butter after removing it from the tandoor.

Real life example

A true socialite, there is rarely a weekend where Swati (name changed) isn't attending some party or a get-together. Having diabetes, she was careful with her food and drink choices. Yet she found that her blood glucose levels would be constantly high.

She came to the clinic to understand why she was finding it difficult to manage her blood glucose levels in spite of having her medication on time and exercising regularly.

During the consultation, she revealed that she had to attend many social events to maintain her social stature. She shared that she had not revealed to anybody other than her immediate family that she has diabetes for the past 3 years.

During such occasions, she consciously stayed away from alcohol and opted for mocktails along with whatever starters were served.

I explained to her that each glass of mocktail had a minimum of 4–5 teaspoons of sugar while almost all the starters were deep-fried and high on carbs. Both these factors were increasing her blood glucose levels. I advised her to choose fresh lime with soda or mojito with plain soda (lots of mint leaves) without sugar. Further, instead of fried starters, I advised her to opt for salad, grilled vegetables and paneer tikka or chicken tandoori.

A tandoori roti without butter or a cup of steamed rice with dal is far more filling and less harmful than a handful of fried snacks. I also advised her to have a bowl of clear soup, buttermilk with some salad or a fruit with a handful of nuts before leaving for the party so that she does not go on a binge.

Healthy Options – Chinese Cuisine

- Steamed rice or noodles
- Steamed dumplings
- All Clear Soups-Mushroom Soup, Steamed Wonton Soup, Lemongrass soup, Chicken or Vegetable Clear soup
- Mixed Vegetables (Mushroom and Bamboo Shoot)
- Stir-Fried Chinese Greens
- Grilled Paneer/Tofu/Chicken/Fish (No Sauce)
- Sautéed Mushrooms with Ginger

- Sautéed Buddhist Vegetable
- Vegetable with Bamboo Fungus
- Stir-fried Chinese Greens Cantonese Style
- Dry Cooked Shanghai Beans with Mushrooms
- Okra, Black Mushroom and Bamboo Shoots with Black bean sauce
- Seasonal Vegetable with broccoli in Chinese Parsley Sauce
- Stir-fried Bean Sprouts with Bell Pepper
- Silken Tofu and Vegetable soup
- Spinach Ginger, Bean curd and Tomato Soup

> Ask for sauces to be served on the side, rather than on the main dish.
>
> Choose Hunan or oyster sauce over a Szechuan sauce.
>
> Choose Stir fry or Sautéed over deep fried

Healthy Options – Mexican & Lebanese Cuisine

- Mexican bowl with kidney beans and fresh salsa
- Grilled/Herbed chicken/fish
- Soft tortillas and beans tacos (not crispy or fried)
- Baked nachos with beans (no cheese)
- Hummus
- Baked falafel

- Burritos
- Gazpacho (tomato) soup
- Moutabbal
- Fatoush (without pita)
- Raheb Salad
- Halloumi
- Guacamole
- Lentils/Lentil Soup
- Tabbouleh

> Ask for grilled vegetables on the side.
>
> Go slow on cheese.

Real life example

Kanika (name changed) is 42 years old and has Type 2 diabetes since the past 7 years. Kanika had a tough time managing her blood glucose levels. Her pre-breakfast blood glucose levels were always above 450 mg/dl and the doctors had advised her to move onto two times a day insulin shots to manage her blood glucose levels.

Kanika came to me for her nutrition consultation. During her consultation she shared that her favourite past time was attending kitty parties. For her and her kitty friends, every new Italian restaurant demanded a try at least once. However, unlike Indian food, Italian dishes are largely served individually and are not typically family-style or sharing dishes. Eating a pizza or pasta with all the additional fat and white sauce was derailing her blood glucose levels.

I gave her a meal plan that was balanced and would help her lower her blood glucose levels. She was asked to avoid eating outside food until her blood glucose levels were absolutely under control. I explained the consequences of eating outside food and its relation to high blood glucose levels.

After a few months of following a healthy eating pattern, exercising regularly, she came back to me happy as her blood glucose levels were almost in the normal range. Only after this, did I allow her to eat her favourite Italian food but only once in a month.

I advised Kanika to eat a small healthy meal at home before heading out. This could be a bowl of salad, nuts, buttermilk, rasam or a bowl of soup, which is nutritious and filling. Further, instead of choosing a double cheese pizza, I advised her to opt for thin crust pizza with lots of vegetables or pasta with tomato sauce or plain pasta tossed in olive oil and vegetables, Spaghetti aglio e olio (garlic spaghetti with less oil). The mini-meal she ate at home stopped her from overindulging at the restaurant while allowing her to enjoy her favourite meal with friends.

If you too are looking for healthy options while enjoying your favourite Italian cuisine, here is the list.

Healthy Options – Italian Cuisine

- Pasta in tomato sauce (arabiata)/marinara sauce (with vegetables in equal proportion) – go slow on the cheese and oil
- Spaghetti aglio e olio(less oil)
- Italian rice with vegetables
- Baked, broiled, grilled, or poached fish/chicken
- Pomodoro salad
- Pasta/Spaghetti (durum wheat) – Bolognese, arabiata, puttalesca, della casa, primavera

- Soups – minestrone, zuppa di broccoli, zuppa di asparagus
- Slim/Cauliflower base pizza (grated cauliflower crust as a base)

You can order a thin crust pizza with tomato sauce, fresh herbs and vegetables, chicken, seafood or turkey. Try and avoid bacon, ham, sausages and pepperoni. Go slow on cheese. Choosing thin crust over thick crust will save you 200 calories per slice of pizza.

> *Avoid items made with cheese and white sauce and cream based soups*

Healthy options – Thai Cuisine

- Steamed rice
- Thai basil chicken
- Tom yum soup (clear soup without coconut milk)
- Satay
- Stir-fried vegetables

Real life example

Sarah (name changed), with her constant battle with high blood glucose levels, chose to switch to south Indian meals whenever she had to eat outside, as she believed it was healthier than other restaurant meals. However, her glucose readings would continue to be high. After visiting a few Udipi restaurants in Mumbai, I found out that many south Indian chains have started mixing maida (refined flour) in their batter to compensate for the rising price of urad dal (lentil). They also add lots of butter and sometimes sugar to make the dosa crispy.

Further, the bowl of sambar is likely to contain sugar or gur (jaggery) added to enhance flavour. These factors affect the blood glucose levels.

Instead, it is better to choose Pessarattu (green gram/moong dal dosa) or Adai, found in authentic south Indian restaurants, as they keep the glucose levels more stable. In case these options are not available on the menu, a tomato omelette or rasam idli are a safe bet.

Sandwiches and Subs

Most people believe that sandwiches & subs is a healthy eating out option. But believe me friends you can eat up to 600 calories in a single sandwich or sub meal. If you add cookies or a soft drink to it then you can swallow up to 1000 calories.

Additionally these calories come from the various fat-laden dressings like mayonnaise, mint mayo, or the extra cheese that cause the blood glucose levels to rise even after a few hours of your meal. While if you know the trick, you can enjoy your meal while managing to control your blood glucose levels.

Always choose whole wheat breads or subs and a generous helping of vegetables.

Healthy options are:

- Veggie Delite sub/sandwich
- Roast Chicken sub/sandwich
- Tuna sub/sandwich

Choose mustard, lemon and vinegar dressing

Real life example

Kunal (name changed) is a 38-year-old marketing head. He was diagnosed with diabetes a few years back. Initially, his blood glucose levels were well controlled but lately they were not well maintained and his recent HbA1c was 9.8%. His doctor changed his medication and asked him to follow a healthy diet. He came to me to seek nutritional advice. On consultation, he shared that he exercises regularly and eats healthy home-cooked food every day. During the consultation, he mentioned that he has to attend many client meetings and has hectic schedules. Most of his meetings were at a coffee shop and he ordered his favourite Café Mocha during these meetings. Café Mocha has chocolate syrup along with sugar and milk which makes it calorie and carb dense.

I suggested that he have Green Tea or Espresso or Cappuccino with low-fat or skimmed milk (without sugar) to see a remarkable change in his blood glucose levels. He followed the advice and his HbA1c over a course of time came down to 7%.

Desserts

It is best to enjoy sweets and desserts only on a special occasion, so that you don't wreck your blood glucose levels. Desserts are made up of refined sugar and can spike your blood glucose levels drastically.

If you need to satisfy your sweet tooth, you can eat a piece of fresh fruit.

However you can enjoy a small piece of birthday cake or a small serving of your favourite dessert once in a while. Count the carbs and make an adjustment to your insulin dosage or make sure you burn the extra calories by working out.

Here are some healthy tips while choosing desserts at restaurants

- Choose a fruit salad instead of a dessert
- If you do want to have a dessert, eat less than half the portion served

- Take advantage of smaller portions available in restaurants or ice cream centres
- Check with the chef if they have any healthy choices in desserts
- Avoid sweets with a lot of cream, or which have been deep-fried

Points to Remember

- What's on your plate will show on your waist.
- Choose wisely and Stay healthy.
- Happy healthy eating out!

Snacking Ideas

Choosing healthy snacks is often a challenge and can be more difficult if you have diabetes. The key is to choose snacks which are nutrient dense- high in fiber, protein and heart-friendly fats. The snacks should help you maintain/lose weight and keep your blood glucose levels under control.

Here are a few snack options you can choose from.

- Plain Yogurt/Curd/Plain Buttermilk
- Handful of Unsalted Nuts and seeds (almonds, walnuts, pistachios, pumpkin seeds, sunflower seeds)
- Vegetable sticks (Raw carrot, beetroot, cucumber, celery stalks) and Hummus/Hung Curd Dip
- Avocado/Guacamole Dip
- Fruit such as apple, pear with Peanut Butter
- Sprouts/Chana Chaat
- Cottage Cheese (paneer) – Grilled/tikka
- Eggs (boiled, omelette, Spanish omelette, egg muffins, poached, scrambled)

- Egg/Chicken/Paneer Salad
- Homemade air-popped popcorn
- Makhana (foxnut)
- Jowar Puffs
- Roasted Chana/Peanuts (unsalted)
- Bhel (Roasted Rice puffs with chana and peanuts)
- Green Gram (moong) khakras
- Sattu (roasted chickpea) flour drink
- Rasam/clear soups.

Healthy Options

You can choose from healthy options that are easily available.

Makhana, also known as Phool Makhana/Fox nut/lotus seeds/Euryale Ferox is a highly nutritious snack. Makhana is very low in saturated fat, and sodium and zero cholesterol. Additionally, it has a low glycemic load, hence recommended for people with diabetes. Makhana is easily available at all grocery stores and supermarkets in most parts of India. Make roasted makhana at home as the ones sold commercially are high in fat and sodium making it unhealthy.

Healthy Snack Recipe – Roasted Makhana

Take 2 cup makhana, ¼ teaspoon turmeric, ½ tsp red chilli powder, rock salt as required and 1 tsp oil or ghee.

Heat oil in a pan or kadai. Add the makhana and roast for 10–12 minutes on a low flame, till they are crisp and crunchy. Keep stirring them in between. Add chilli powder, turmeric powder and salt. Switch off the flame and stir the mixture well.

Once they cool down, store roasted makhana in an airtight container.

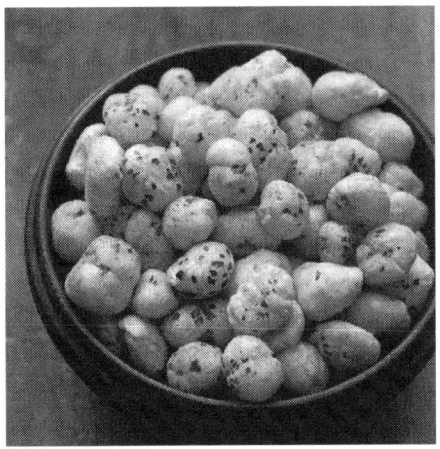

Healthy Snack Recipe – Soy nuts

Ingredient: 1 cup soya bean, ¼ tsp chilli powder, ¼ tsp turmeric powder salt as required.

Soak soya bean overnight. Sundry it the next day. Heat a pan or kadai. Add dried soya bean and salt. Roast it for 10–15minutes on a low flame till they become crisp. Keep stirring them in between. Add red chilli powder and turmeric powder (optional). Switch off the flame and stir the mixture well. Once they cool down store the mixture in an airtight container.

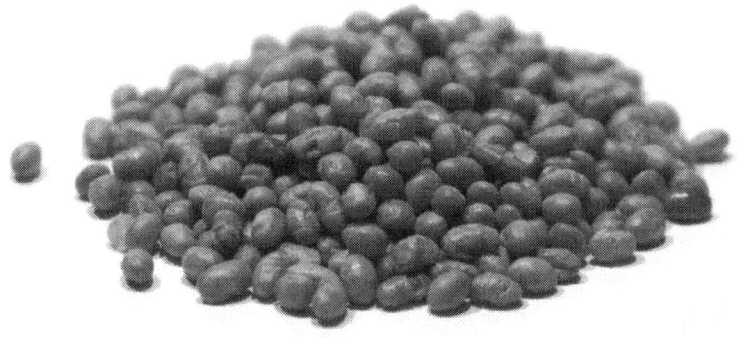

CHAPTER 15

Smart Cooking

Authored by Natasha Vora
(Msc Foods, Nutrition and Dietetics, CDE)

Cooking is a culinary art which transforms basic food ingredients into palatable and wholesome meals. It improves food digestibility, increases the availability of some nutrients and decreases anti-nutritional factors. However, did you know that some nutrients are lost in the process of cooking? During preparation or actual cooking of food, exposure to heat, light, and oxygen alter the nutrients in the food which may lead to significant nutrient losses. This chapter will help you understand the critical processes when nutrients might be lost during preparation and cooking. It will help you develop the art of smart cooking to be able to enjoy delicious and nutritious food.

Effects of preparation and cooking methods on food:

Washing: Water-soluble vitamins like B complex vitamins and Vitamin C are easily lost when vegetables containing them are washed. Repeated washing of food grains like rice and pulses results in a loss of valuable minerals and vitamins.

> Do not wash food grains repeatedly before cooking.
>
> Wash vegetables well before cutting them as washing cut vegetables leads to greater loss of nutrients as more of the nutrients are exposed to water.

Soaking: Soaking grains and pulses is a traditional practice that has a positive impact on the nutritional qualities of these foods. While these foods add variety to your diet, they contain certain anti-nutritional factors which do not allow proteins to be digested properly and reduce the availability of certain minerals. Soaking helps reduce anti-nutritional factors like phytates, tannins and enzyme inhibitors thus increasing absorption value of nutrients from these foods.

> *Pulses and grains should be soaked and cooked to increase the nutrient availability from them to meet the protein and mineral requirements.*

Boiling: Boiling refers to cooking food in water boiling at 100°C. Although this method is quick and easy, the large volume of water dissolves and washes away water-soluble vitamins including 60 to 70 percent of foods' minerals. Vitamin C, being water-soluble and sensitive to heat, leaches into the hot water when it is boiled. In fact, boiling reduces vitamin C more than any other cooking method. Broccoli, spinach and lettuce may lose up to 50% or more of vitamin C when boiled. Vitamin B like Thiamin(B1), Folate, and vitamin B 12 are easily destroyed by heat. Vitamin B12 deficiency is quite common in India which is why it is necessary to preserve these vital nutrients. The good news is that when it comes to Omega-3 fatty acids, research shows that boiling fish preserves the heart-friendly Omega-3 fatty acids much more as compared to frying fish. You also save on calories that way!

> *If you choose to boil your food, make sure you retain the water and use it to make gravies, soups or to knead the dough. This way you retain 100% of the minerals and 70–90% of B vitamins.*
>
> *Use minimum water while cooking, just enough to cook.*

> Root vegetables like potato, sweet potato, colocasia (arbi), suran, etc. should be boiled with their skins. This helps the nutrients to move to the centre of the vegetable, thereby helping better retention of nutrients.
>
> When boiling, let the water boil first and then add the raw vegetables.

Steaming: Steaming is one of the best cooking methods for preserving nutrients, including water-soluble vitamins that are sensitive to heat and water. Studies have shown that steaming is the best method to preserve the nutritional quality of broccoli and its anti-cancer phytonutrients. Vitamin C and vitamin B losses are the least by this method of cooking.

> Steam or pressure cook your vegetables with minimum water instead of boiling them. This way you preserve maximum nutrients.

Grilling and Roasting: Opt for these methods when you want to lower your fat consumption as they are dry heat cooking methods. However as they involve high heat there are losses of heat-sensitive vitamins and minerals. Since grilling is a common method when it comes to non-vegetarian food like fish and meat, there is a concern of overproduction of Polycyclic Aromatic Hydrocarbons (PAHs), which are chemicals formed when meat is cooked directly over open flame. These chemicals are found to be carcinogenic (cancer-causing). The most important factor contributing to the production of PAHs in grilling is smoke resulting from incomplete combustion of fat dripped onto the fire.

> Just stick to lean cuts of meat that require less cooking time and have lower fat content to lower the production of PAHs.

Real life example

Reya (name changed) adds a lot of seeds to her daily meals as they are nutritious. She adds flaxseed powder to her raita, flakes, salad etc. She generally roasts the flaxseeds at home and then grinds it to powder form and stores it in an airtight container. The most common mistake that many people including Reya do is roasting flaxseeds on a hot griddle/tawa after making chapattis.

The problem here is that flaxseeds contain Omega-3 fatty acids which are easily degraded when exposed to excessive heat. Omega-3 fatty acids are very important for people with diabetes as they help to improve good cholesterol levels and reduce triglycerides, thus lowering the risk of heart disease which is a common complication of diabetes.

So what's the right way to eat flaxseeds? Lightly roast the seeds (heat the pan and switch off the flame). Powder the seeds and consume the powder.

Microwave Cooking: The invention of the microwave has been a boon for those who are pressed for time. A lot of debate with contrasting views on whether microwave cooking is safe or not has been carried on for a long time. Most of the studies have shown that microwave cooking is a safe and convenient mode of cooking.

> *Make sure you use only "Microwave safe" containers (No Plastic) to cook the food.*

Sautéing and Stir-Frying: These are cooking methods in which food is cooked in a saucepan over medium to high heat in a small amount of oil or butter. In general, this is a healthy way to prepare food. It involves shorter cooking time without water which prevents loss of B vitamins. Since this method involves high heat, it is detrimental to vitamin C. However, the advantage of this type of cooking is that it involves the addition of some fat which enables better absorption of the fat-soluble vitamins and antioxidants.

Use these methods of cooking to improve absorption of fat soluble vitamins.

Keep cooking time to minimum to preserve maximum nutrients.

Fermentation: Fermentation is a process in which microorganisms feed on the sugar and starch in the food creating lactic acid and carbon dioxide. Commonly consumed fermented foods in India are idli, dosa, dhokla, curd and cheese. This process preserves the food, and creates beneficial enzymes which help in digestion. This method of processing food also helps to generate live "good" bacteria called probiotics. Probiotics help to maintain gut health and improve immunity. In the process of fermentation of milk into curd, lactose gets converted to lactic acid and simpler sugars which can be digested even if you are lactose intolerant. Fermentation of pulses helps to reduce anti-nutritional factors such as phytic acid which is broken down during fermentation, so the minerals become more available. Overnight fermentation of idli batter increases the vitamin B and C in the batter. The reported changes during fermentation include an increase in free sugar due to which the Glycemic Index (GI) of fermented foods like idli or dosa increases. So for a person with diabetes, fermented foods can cause an increase in blood glucose levels which can be prevented by consuming fermented foods along with good fibre intake like vegetables or salads to reduce the GI of the meal.

Fermented foods increase nutrient availability but should be consumed with high fiber foods to reduce GI

Frying: This method involves cooking food in a large amount of oil at high temperatures. Frying is not recommended often due to excess fat intake contributing to excess calorie intake leading to obesity. Frying has little or no impact on the protein or mineral content of fried food. Moreover, the short time of the frying process causes less loss of heat liable vitamins. However, research shows that it degrades the Omega-3 content of food by 70–85%. Also, one needs to be careful as to which oil is used for frying.

When oil is heated past its smoke point, (the point at which bluish smoke emerges from oil) it generates toxic fumes and free radicals which are extremely harmful to your body. Hence oil with low smoking points such as olive oil and flaxseed oil should not be used for frying foods. When the oil is heated to a high temperature for a long period of time, toxic substances called aldehydes are formed. Aldehydes have been linked to an increased risk of cancer and other neurodegenerative diseases. Hence oil once used for frying should never be reused for frying. Reusing the oil for frying also leads to the formation of trans-fat which increases the risk to heart diseases.

Use of air fryer: Recent invention of the air fryer has made a revolution in the consumer's mind about enjoying their favourite foods without the intake of the biggest villain 'oil'. Air fryers use swirling hot air to create the crispy, browned texture that you get from deep-fried foods, but with only a fraction of the oil. Although there are very few studies on the effect of this method of cooking on nutrients, its advantage is that it provides quick cooking and results similar to the typically deep fat fried food but with controlled oil content. So an air fryer can be used as a substitute to deep frying provided it is not used as an excuse to eat unhealthy foods like fries often while skipping on healthy food like vegetables!

> Use frying sparingly, as a method of cooking.
>
> Do not use oils with low smoking point for frying.
>
> Oil once used for frying should not be reused again for frying. It can be used for tempering.
>
> Air fryers can be used as a substitute but only occasionally.

In addition to these common cooking methods, there are several other factors that can lead to a loss of nutrients. These are:

Air: Exposure to air, basically oxygen causes oxidation of Vitamin C. Oxidative losses increase with temperature, long cooking time and cutting vegetables into small pieces or mashing them. Vitamin A is also prone to oxidation.

> Cut salads just before you are going to serve them.
>
> Serve salads and gravies in closed dishes to avoid exposure to air.
>
> Do not cut vegetables into very small pieces as each small part will come in contact with oxygen thus destroying the vitamins.
>
> Fruits should be cut just before serving to save the Vitamin C.

Light: Vitamins such as Riboflavin (Vitamin B2), vitamin E and K are light sensitive. Sun-drying and cooking foods in pots open to light destroy these vitamins.

> Keep food covered at all times.

Alkaline medium: Adding cooking soda (sodium bicarbonate) while preparing food, makes the cooking medium alkaline. It enhances the colour of green vegetables, and fastens the cooking process. However, it destroys vitamin B 1, B2, B6, vitamin C and vitamin K to a large extent.

The bottom line is that there is no perfect method of cooking that retains all the nutrients but it's important to select the right cooking method to maximize the nutritional quality of your meal. The thumb rule is:

> Keep cooking time, temperature, and the amount of liquid to a minimum.

Reduce your AGE

Yes, if you want your mind and body to remain young, reduce your AGE consumption from foods. Advanced glycation end products (AGEs) naturally form inside the body when proteins or fats combine with sugars (glycation). This affects the normal functioning of cells, making them more susceptible to damage and premature ageing. In addition to AGEs that form within the body, AGEs also exist in foods. They contribute to increased oxidative stress and inflammation which increases the risk of diabetes, heart disease, kidney disease, Alzheimer's and premature ageing. People with diabetes need to be more careful as they are anyways at a higher risk for producing too many AGEs.

The most effective way to reduce AGEs in food is to modify cooking methods. Cooking methods which use high temperatures to brown or char foods, such as grilling, roasting, baking, frying, broiling, toasting have the largest impact on the amount of AGEs consumed. In fact, dry heat causes AGE formation to increase by 10 to 100 times than the levels in uncooked foods.

Tips to lower AGE consumption from food

- Prefer moist cooking methods like stewing, poaching, boiling and steaming over dry cooking.

- Cook with moist heat, at lower temperature and for a shorter span of time.

- Marinate foods in acidic ingredients, such as vinegar, tomato juice or lemon juice. This can reduce AGE production by up to 50%.

- Try to avoid animal foods like red meat, processed meat and other highly processed and sugary foods that have high AGE's and instead choose natural foods like fruits, vegetables and whole grains which have lower AGE even after cooking.

Reheating Food

There are very few opportunities where you eat food that is freshly prepared and served right out of the pan. In this era where everyone has busy schedules, food is cooked well in advance. It is carried in tiffin/dabbas to the office or school for lunch. In houses with working women, dinner is prepared in the morning and stored in the refrigerator to be reheated later at night. This is not a healthy practice for certain foods.

There are some food items which are healthy but can lose their nutrients when reheated. For instance, **Spinach and Beetroot** contain nitrates in high concentration. When you reheat beetroot/spinach, nitrates get converted to nitrites. Nitrites can affect the oxygen level in the blood; they have carcinogenic properties (cancer-causing) and can cause food poisoning when reheated.

Did You Know?

Tips to get the best out of your food

Sprouting pulses increases Vitamin C content and some B-group Vitamins.

Lycopene, found in tomatoes is a powerful antioxidant. Heating or pureeing tomatoes makes the lycopene more available for absorption and so cooked tomatoes provide better anti-cancer effect.

Onions should be cooked or baked to improve antioxidant content.

Health benefits from garlic are best obtained by chopping or crushing it and letting it sit before heating it along with other recipe ingredients.

Cooking in iron utensils increases the total as well as the available iron content of the food.

Resistant starch–a form of starch which remains undigested, is formed when starch-containing foods are cooked and cooled, such as legumes, bread, rice, corn, potatoes, pasta. This helps to lower the glycemic index of food and blunts the blood glucose response. So for better blood glucose control, cook these foods a day prior, refrigerate and consume them the next day without reheating them to high temperatures.

CHAPTER 16 Superfoods

As rightly said by the father of medicine, Hippocrates, "Let food be thy medicine and medicine be thy food"

Here are some inexpensive and easy to find foods from the kitchen which have shown immense benefits in improving blood glucose levels in patients with diabetes.

Amla (Indian Gooseberry)

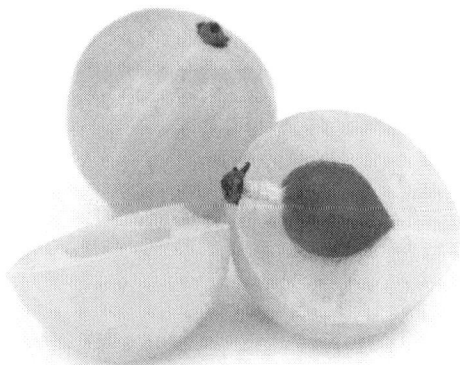

Amla, also known as the Indian Gooseberry, is the richest source of vitamin C and is packed with many other vitamins and minerals. Vitamin C in 1 amla is equal to vitamin C in 2 oranges. Amla has also shown to be effective in controlling blood glucose and blood cholesterol levels. Dried amla is as good as fresh amla as it contains substances which partially protect the vitamin C from destruction on heating or drying.

How to consume:

Amla can be consumed as the fruit itself or as fresh amla juice or amla powder.

Recommended Dosage:

One to three grams of amla powder daily.

Rajma (Kidney Beans)

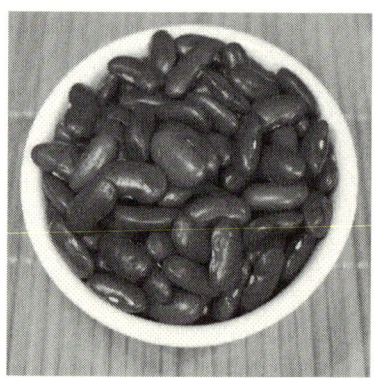

Kidney beans are a very good source of cholesterol-lowering fibre, as are most other beans. In addition to lowering cholesterol, kidney beans' high fibre content prevents blood glucose levels from rising too rapidly after a meal, making these beans an especially good choice for individuals with diabetes and insulin resistance. Rajma rice is everyone's favourite. Isn't it? When combined with whole grains such as rice, kidney beans provide virtually fat-free high-quality protein while helping you balance blood glucose levels.

How to consume:

Kidney beans can be eaten with rice (Rajmah chawal) or can be added to salads, soups, tikkis or gravy.

Recommended Dosage:

Include 3 bowls of cooked rajma a week to enjoy its health benefits.

Sweet potatoes

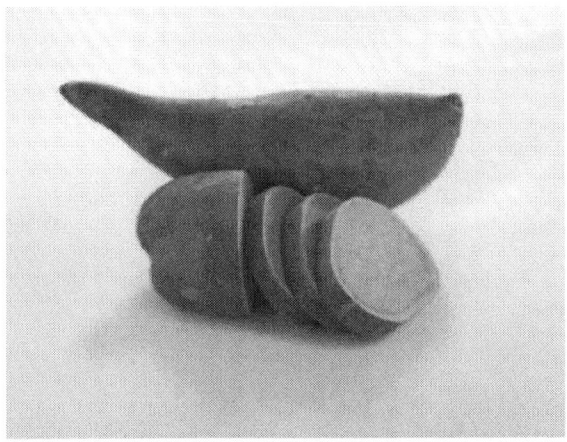

Sweet potatoes can be a good choice for patients with diabetes as they are a good source of fibre and have a moderate glycemic index. Consuming sweet potatoes with skin adds to the fiber content and gives a feeling of satiety.

Sweet Potatoes are a good post work out snacking option. The carbs are great for replenishing your glycogen stores (stored carbs) after an intense bout of exercise. To make this post-workout snack complete, eat your sweet potato with a good source of lean protein like paneer, yogurt or a piece of grilled chicken or boiled egg whites.

They have also shown to reduce "bad" LDL cholesterol in the body due to its fiber content. Ensure to have it in moderation after consultation with your dietitian and doctor.

Soybean

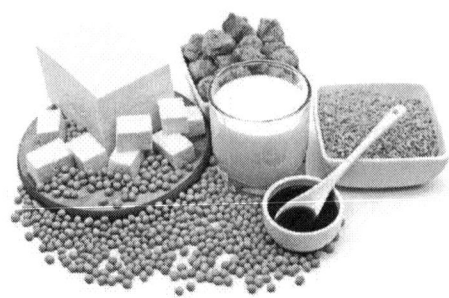

Soybean is a boon to vegetarians as it is a rich source of protein (20gms soybean has 7 grams of protein). It is also a good source of calcium, iron, phytoestrogens and the heart-friendly omega – 3 fatty acids. Soybean scores over animal products and milk as it is cholesterol and lactose-free and can be given to people with lactose intolerance. It can also be given to people with gluten intolerance.

The beneficial effects of soy in regulating blood glucose levels are attributed to isoflavones which are present in soy beans. Isoflavones help to increase insulin secretion, thereby improving blood glucose control. Soybean helps to lower not only glucose levels in the blood but also is beneficial in reducing blood cholesterol levels.

Studies have shown that including 40 g of soy protein in the diet can help increase bone mineral density thereby preventing osteoporosis.

How to consume:

Soybean can be incorporated easily in our daily meal plan in the form of unflavoured soy milk, soy paneer/cheese (tofu), soy granules (nutrela and nuggets), soy atta, soy yogurt, and soy nuts are available freely at all supermarkets and at many grocery stores

Soya should be roasted/cooked before use to destroy the anti-nutritional properties!

Flaxseeds

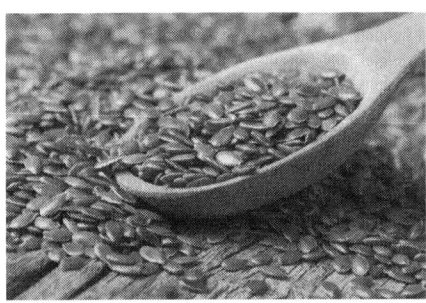

Several studies have shown that flax seeds help in lowering triglyceride levels and stabilizing blood glucose levels. Flaxseeds contain 7.6 grams of fibre/28grams (1 ounce) and are a rich source of Omega-3 fatty acids. They contain both insoluble and soluble fibre which helps to lower cholesterol and triglyceride levels in the blood.

Flaxseeds have a thick husk that cannot be digested, so they must be ground for your body to get its nutritional benefits. Roast the flax seeds on a low flame before grinding. Store them in a dark, cool place to prevent them from getting rancid.

How to consume:

Add a tablespoon of ground flaxseeds to your breakfast cereal/smoothie/yoghurt/salads/baked foods.

Recommended Dosage:

1 tbsp of powdered flaxseed per day.

Avoid consuming in large amounts as it can have adverse health effects

Barley

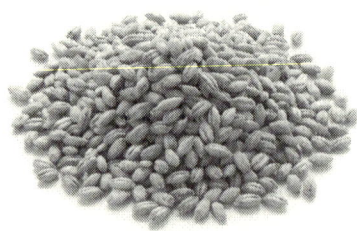

Barley is an excellent food choice for those with diabetes or pre-diabetes because the grain contains essential vitamins and minerals and is an excellent source of dietary fibre, particularly soluble fibre. Unlike many grains which contain fibre only in the outer bran layer, barley contains fibre throughout the entire kernel. So whether it's whole grain or processed barley products, dietary fibre, including beta-glucan soluble fibre, is available in amounts that have a positive impact in improving blood glucose levels.

How to consume:

As a grain in soups/khichdi/salads or flour to make rotis/pancakes/khakra

Recommended Dosage:

1.5 cups of cooked barley give adequate fibre for health benefit

Fenugreek seeds

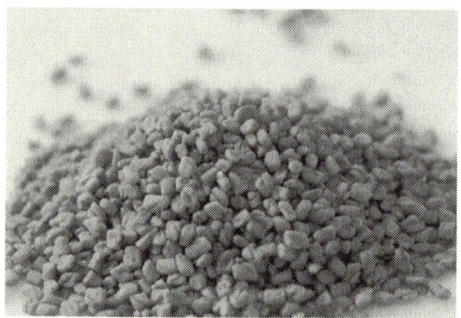

Fenugreek (methi) is known to be an effective home remedy for controlling blood glucose levels. The sugar lowering property of fenugreek seeds is attributed to the presence of soluble fibre, which not only reduces the rate of digestion by the enzymes but also reduces the absorption of glucose from the stomach. These seeds also contain trigonelline, a compound which reduces glucose levels in the blood. Moreover, the presence of 4-hydroxyisoleucine, a novel amino acid, in fenugreek stimulates glucose-dependent insulin release by the pancreatic cells thereby helping you to control your blood glucose naturally.

Fenugreek seeds are also packed with polyphenols and flavonoids which exert antioxidant action thus lowering cholesterol and triglyceride levels in the body. The fibre galactomannan exerts lipid (blood fat) lowering effect by forming a viscous gel in the intestine and hence, limits the absorption of fat and glucose.

How to consume:

- Methi seed powder can be incorporated in chapatti flour
- Sprouted Methi can be added to Salads
- Methi can be added to milk while setting curds
- Can be consumed after overnight soaking in water or in a powder form as a drink in water or buttermilk first thing in the morning or 15 minutes before meals

Recommended Dosage:

15–30 gm (1–2 tbsp) per day

Cinnamon (*Dalchini*)

Cinnamon is a superfood offering great health benefits. Studies have shown that it helps regulate blood glucose levels, boost metabolism thus helping in weight loss, offers heart protective benefits by lowering blood pressure and cholesterol levels. It also helps improve immunity due to its antioxidant property

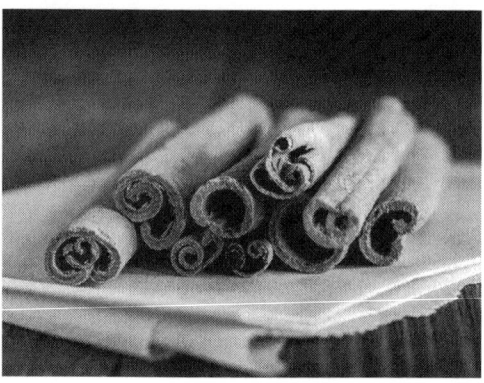

How to consume:

Freshly pounded cinnamon can be added to water, green tea, porridge, cut fruits. Ensure you buy the ceylon cinnamon

Recommended Dosage:

½-1 tsp of freshly pounded cinnamon powder per day

Avoid consuming in large amounts as it can have adverse health effects

Apple Cider Vinegar

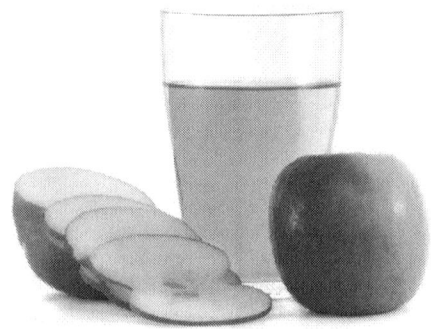

Apple cider vinegar, a health tonic is found to be beneficial for treating allergies, acidity, aiding in digestion and promoting weight loss. The American Diabetes Association recommends apple cider vinegar as a way to help insulin work better and improve blood glucose control. Studies have shown that apple cider vinegar when consumed with water showed a reduction in LDL (bad) cholesterol. Because of its strong flavour and relatively low caloric content, apple cider vinegar is a healthy alternative to creamy dressings and sauces.

How to consume:

- Can be diluted in water and taken before meals or at bedtime to reduce fasting blood glucose.
- Can be used as a salad dressing.

Recommended Dosage:

10 ml ACV (unfiltered and with the mother) with a glass of water to be taken 15 minutes before meals or at bedtime

Ispaghula husk (psyllium/isabgol)

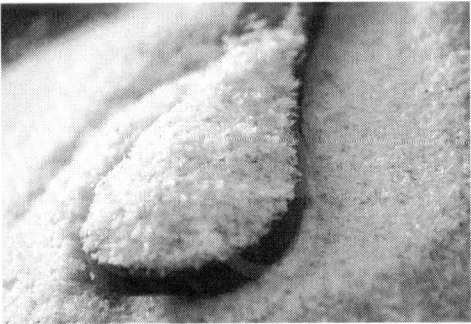

Psyllium (husk) is a soluble fibre used primarily as a gentle bulk-forming laxative. It has also shown to aid weight loss, provide satiety and lower blood glucose levels. Studies have shown that 5 gram of psyllium twice a day causes an approx. 5% reduction in total serum cholesterol and

7% reduction in LDL (bad) cholesterol. If Psyllium is taken before meals, it lowers post-meal blood glucose levels by 15–20%. Psyllium increases the feeling of fullness and reduces hunger craving thereby help in weight reduction.

Recommended Dosage:

- The recommended daily intake for fibre is 25 grams to 35 grams per day.
- One to three teaspoon a day to be taken with adequate water.

CHAPTER 17 Healthy Recipes
===

Authored by Shweta Gosalia (RD,CDE)

Broccoli and sweet potato salad

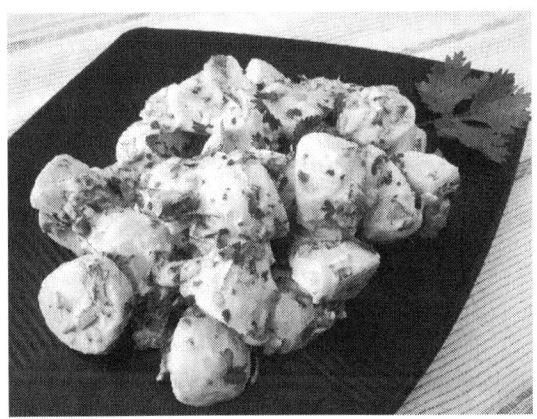

Serves: 2

Ingredients	Amounts
Small Broccoli Florets(steamed)	1 cup
**Sweet potato cubes (Cooked and cooled)	1 cup
Toasted walnuts (roughly chopped)	1 tbsp
For Dressing	
Hung Curd	½ cup
Garlic-green chilli paste	¼ tsp

Salt	To taste
Pepper	¼ tsp
Cumin powder (Roasted)	¼ tsp

*1 cup = 200 ml   *1 tbsp = 15 ml   *1 tsp = 5 ml

Method for preparing Dressing:

Mix together all of the above ingredients for the dressing and refrigerate for 30 minutes.

Method for preparing Salad:

- Mix the broccoli and sweet potatoes together gently.
- Cover and refrigerate for 30 minutes and then toss with the cold dressing.
- Garnish with toasted walnuts.

**Boil sweet potato one day prior. Cool in the refrigerator for 24 hours and use the next day. Do not reheat at high temperature.

Nutritive value per serving:

Energy (Kcal)	Proteins (g)	Carbohydrates (g)	Fats (g)
186	6.8	23	7.5

Buckwheat Dhokla

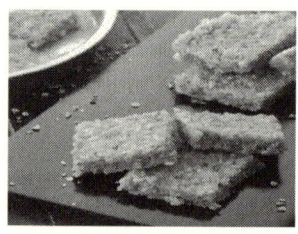

Serves: 1 (Makes – 5 to 6 pieces)

Ingredients	Amounts
Buckwheat (Kuttu)	½ cup
Buttermilk	½ cup
Ginger-green chilli paste	½ tsp
Salt	to taste
Fruit salt	a pinch
Oil for greasing	¼ tsp

*1 cup = 200 ml   *1 tbsp = 15 ml   *1 tsp = 5 ml

Method:

- Clean and wash buckwheat with water. Drain the excess water using a strainer.
- Combine the buckwheat and buttermilk in a bowl and mix well. Cover with a lid and keep aside to soak for to 6 to 7 hours.
- Add the ginger-green chilli paste and salt to the mixture and mix well to make the dhokla batter.
- Add the fruit salt to the batter and sprinkle a little water over it to enable bubbles to be formed.
- Mix gently and pour the batter into a 200 mm/(8") diameter greased thali.
- Steam for 10 to 12 minutes till the dhoklas are firm.
- Cool slightly and cut into diamond-shaped pieces.
- Serve hot with coriander and mint chutney.

Nutritive value per serving:

Energy (Kcal)	Proteins (g)	Carbohydrates (g)	Fats (g)
162	5.6	28	3.1

Egg Appams

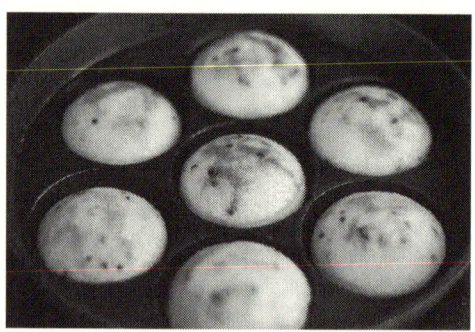

Serves: 1 (Makes 6 to 8 Appams)

Ingredients	Amounts
Egg whites	4 no.
American Corn, boiled	½ cup
Bell peppers (yellow and red), cubes	½ cup
Tomatoes, chopped	2 tbsp
Italian herb seasoning	To Taste
Oil	1 tsp
Salt	To Taste
Black Olives, sliced	For garnish

*1 cup = 200 ml   *1 tbsp = 15 ml   *1 tsp = 5 ml

Method:

- Take a pan, add 1 tsp of oil. Add tomatoes, American corn, bell peppers, Italian seasoning and salt and sauté for 2 minutes. Turn off the gas immediately. Keep it aside.
- Take a paniyaram pan. Heat it and grease it with little oil.
- Put the prepared stuffing in each paniyaram holder and then top it up with the egg whites.

- Cook it on a low flame for 8 to 10 minutes. Remove it and garnish it with sliced olives on each appam.

Nutritive value per serving:

Energy (Kcal)	Proteins (g)	Carbohydrates (g)	Fats (g)
158	14.0	13.0	5.6

Foxtail Millet (Navane) Pulav

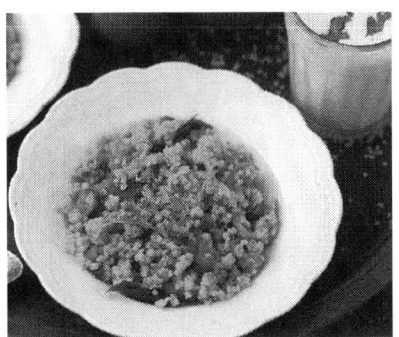

Serves: 2

Ingredients	Amounts
Ghee	2 tsp
Cumin seeds	¼ tsp
Green chilli, slit	1 no.
Small onion, thinly sliced	1 no.
Ginger, peeled and finely chopped	1 inch pc
Curry leaves, optional	A few
Turmeric	¼ tsp
Diced carrots	¼ cup
Shelled green peas	½ cup
Foxtail Millet (Navane)	½ cup

Salt	To taste
Chopped cilantro/Coriander	for garnish

*1 cup = 200 ml   *1 tbsp = 15 ml   *1 tsp = 5 ml

Method:

- In a large saucepan, heat the ghee and add the cumin seeds. When they sizzle, add the green chilli, onions, ginger and curry leaf. Stir on medium heat till the onion is soft and translucent.

- Now add the turmeric, carrots, and peas. Stir while cooking for about a minute.

- Add the foxtail millets to the saucepan and stir gently for a few seconds. Then pour in 4 cups water and salt and bring to a boil. Reduce heat to low, and simmer covered till all the water is absorbed and the foxtail is cooked, about 15 minutes.

- Serve hot, garnished with chopped cilantro/coriander.

Nutritive value per serving:

Energy (Kcal)	Proteins (g)	Carbohydrates (g)	Fats (g)
220	7.1	32.2	7.0

Makhana (Foxnut) Paneer Chaat

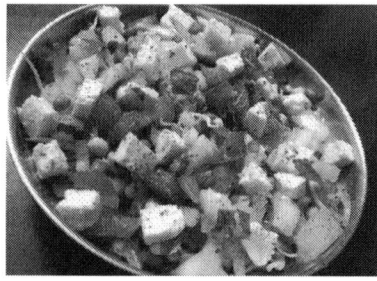

Serves: 2

Ingredients	Amounts
Roasted Makhana/Fox nut	1 cup
Paneer	½ cup
Sprouts (Optional)	½ cup
Tomato diced	½ cup
Cucumber diced	½ cup
Chopped coriander	1 tbsp
Lemon juice	1 tbsp
Black pepper powder	¼ tsp
Salt to taste	1 tsp

*1 cup = 200 ml   *1 tbsp = 15 ml   *1 tsp = 5 ml

Method:

Mix paneer, tomatoes, cucumber and coriander in a large bowl. Add Makhana, Sprouts, lemon juice, salt and pepper to it. Toss and serve well.

Nutritive value per serving:

Energy (Kcal)	Proteins (g)	Carbohydrates (g)	Fats (g)
190	10	15	10

Nourishing Barley soup

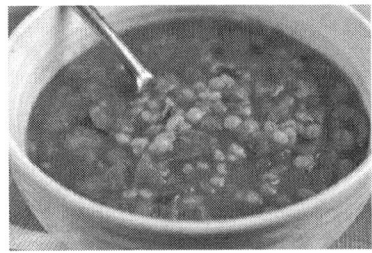

Serves: 2

Ingredients	Amount
Pearl Barley (Soaked for 3–4 hours)	1/3 cup
Whole masoor (Soaked overnight and drained)	½ cup
Garlic clove, chopped	1 clove
Spring onions (finely chopped)-Greens and white separated	½ cup
Carrots, diced	½ cup
Tomatoes, chopped	½ cup
Coriander, chopped	For garnishing
Oil	1 tsp
Salt and Pepper	To taste

*1 cup = 200 ml   *1 tbsp = 15 ml   *1 tsp = 5 ml

Method:

- Drain soaked barley and keep aside.
- Heat oil in a pressure cooker; add the garlic and spring onions (white) and sauté till the onion whites turn translucent.
- Add barley, masoor, carrots, salt and 2 ½ cups of water and pressure cook for 3–4 whistles. Cool slightly.
- Add the spring onion (greens), tomatoes, coriander and pepper and bring it to a boil. Serve hot.

Nutritive value per serving:

Energy (Kcal)	Proteins (g)	Carbohydrates (g)	Fats (g)
103	4.3	15	3.0

Nutribowl-One Pot Meal

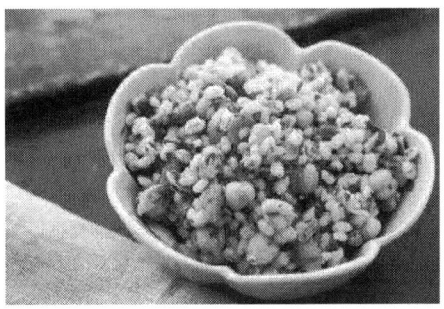

Serves: 2

Ingredients	Amounts
Boiled Barley	½ cup
Boiled chickpeas	½ cup
Paneer	100 g
Tomato diced	1 cup
Bell peppers diced	1 cup
Chopped coriander	½ cup
Salt	To taste
For Dressing	
Extra Virgin Olive oil	2 tsp
Lemon juice	2 tsp (juice of half lemon)
Mixed herbs	As per taste
Black pepper powder	¼ tsp

*1 cup = 200 ml   *1 tbsp = 15 ml   *1 tsp = 5 ml

Method:

- In a large mixing bowl, add boiled barley, boiled chickpeas, scrambled paneer, bell peppers, diced tomatoes, seed mix, chopped coriander leaves. Mix well.

- Add salt as per taste.
- Prepare a dressing using lemon juice, Extra Virgin olive oil, black pepper powder and herbs.
- Pour over the above mixture, mix well and serve.

Nutritive value per serving:

Energy (Kcal)	Proteins (g)	Carbohydrates (g)	Fats (g)
276	13.5	22.5	15

Palak Rajmah Wrap

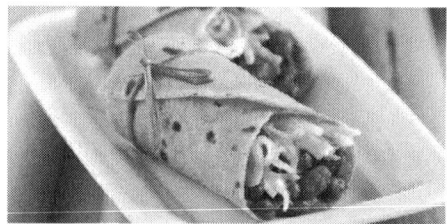

Serves: 1

Ingredients	Amounts
Rajma, soaked overnight and boiled	½ cup
Spinach, chopped	½ cup
Chapattis, whole wheat	1 no.
Onion, diced	1 no.
Lettuce leaf (shredded)	1 no.
Oil	1 tsp
Hung curd	2 tbsp
Garlic clove, minced	2 no.

Chilli powder	1 tbsp
Fresh tomatoes, chopped	1 cup
Ground cumin	1 tsp
Tomato salsa	1 tbsp
Salt	To taste

*1 cup = 200 ml   *1 tbsp = 15 ml   *1 tsp = 5 ml

Method:

- Heat oil in a large frying pan on medium-high heat.
- Sauté onion and garlic for 5 minutes.
- Stir in chilli powder and cumin, and cook 1 minute.
- Stir in tomato, rajma and salt. Bring to the boil, then reduce heat and simmer for 10 minutes.
- Stir in spinach and cook 5 minutes more.
- Remove from heat. Cool it for 10 minutes.
- Spoon 1/2 of the mixture into the middle of a warm chapatti.
- Top it up with lettuce (shredded), hung curd and salsa.
- Wrap it and serve!

Nutritive value per serving:

Energy (Kcal)	Proteins (g)	Carbohydrates (g)	Fats (g)
227	7.0	33	7.5

Chana dal and Cabbage Tikki

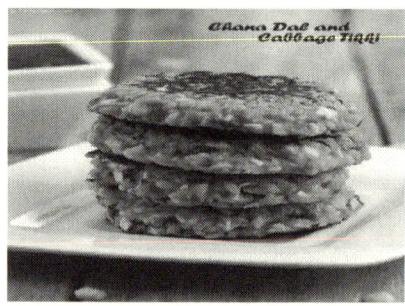

Serves: 1 (Makes 4)

Ingredients	Amounts
Chana dal (soaked for 6 to 8 hours)	½ cup
Cabbage (chopped)	½ cup
Green chilly	1 no.
Mint leaves (chopped)	2 tbsp
Turmeric powder	¼ tsp
Cumin seeds powder	½ tsp
Curd	1 tbsp.
Gram Flour (Besan)	1 tbsp
Salt	To taste
Oil	1 tsp.

*1 cup = 200 ml   *1 tbsp = 15 ml   *1 tsp = 5 ml

Method:

- Combine the Chana dal, green chillies and 2 tbsp of water in a mixer and blend in a mixer to a coarse paste.

- Transfer the paste into a bowl, add all the remaining ingredients and mix well.

- Divide the mixture into 4 equal portions and keep aside.
- Heat a non-stick tava and grease it using 1/4 tsp of oil.
- Shape the mixture into flat round tikkis and immediately cook it on the tava on a slow flame. add the remaining oil and cook all the tikkis till they turn golden brown in colour from both the sides.
- Serve hot with mint and coriander chutney.

Nutritive value per serving:

Energy (Kcal)	Proteins (g)	Carbohydrates (g)	Fats (g)
193	8.7	24.0	7.0

Broken Wheat Pulav

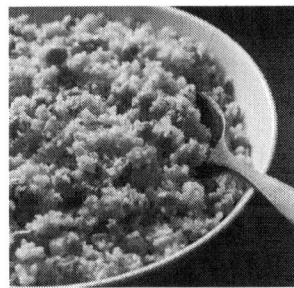

Serves: 2

Ingredients	Amounts
Broken wheat (Daliya)	½ cup
Soy chunks	½ cup
Onions (chopped)	¼ cup
Carrots (chopped)	¼ cup
Capsicum (chopped)	¼ cup
Cabbage	¼ cup

Oil	1 tsp
Cumin seeds	¼ tsp
Bay leaves	1–2 no.
Green chilli	1 (cut length wise)
Ginger-Garlic paste	¼ tsp
Clove-cinnamon stick	1 each
Garam masala	1 tsp
Salt	To taste

*1 cup = 200 ml   *1 tbsp = 15 ml   *1 tsp = 5 ml

Method:

- Heat oil in a pressure pan and splutter cumin seeds. Add Bay leaves, green chilli, clove and cinnamon stick.
- Add onions and sauté for one minute. Add Ginger garlic paste.
- Add all the vegetables and sauté for 2 to 3 minutes and then add soy nuggets.
- Add the broken wheat (soaked for half an hour) and saute for 5 minutes.
- Add 2 ½ cups of water, salt and garam masala.
- Close the lid and cook for 3 whistles.
- Serve Hot with curd.

Nutritive value per serving:

Energy (Kcal)	Proteins (g)	Carbohydrates (g)	Fats (g)
178	9.0	22.0	6.0

Testimonials

Here are a few testimonials from our patrons. The love we receive from them and faith they have in us motivates us to do better work.

I met Sheryl through my doctor in April 2012. I was on the pump then and just found out I was pregnant. Since then my only aim in life was to have well controlled sugar levels and maintain my HbA1c to level 6 or below throughout my pregnancy because I knew the importance of good sugars or the disadvantages of bad sugars on my pregnancy and twin babies. I was worried as it meant I had to control the food I was eating. But thanks to Sheryl, I achieved my goal. She was there at any time of the day, and also the night. For her literally her patients are most important I feel. And the best part about her is, she never says no for anything you feel like eating. Even if I felt like having anything like fries, she would say no problem. Go ahead, but just have so much and take the X amt of units. And trust me I was happy about even that. Most dietitians would stop you from eating certain kinds of food, obviously for our good but they don't understand the human mind where, the more you stop someone from doing a certain thing, the more the desire. And Sheryl very well knew how to manage that. She builds such a lovely relationship with her patients that over a period of time she becomes a friend more than anything. She was even there for me from 12.30am onwards during my labour guiding my husband how frequently to keep a check on my sugars and to make me have sugar water, just so that I don't go into hypoglycaemia. She is a very caring and a very warm person to interact with. So you would never feel awkward asking/telling her anything. We love her and feel blessed to have her in our life. And I would definitely recommend her to anyone who would want to improve their sugar levels and have a healthy lifestyle

– Dr. Miraya Mangtani,
Doctor and Mother of Twins, Dubai

Sheryl – the God of diabetes educators and above all who cares for you. (gives personal attention ~approachable 24/7).

If one has diabetes, you must know Sheryl.

My name is Manish Lakhi. For some reason, God did not only want to see me as a a person with diabetes but made me one unique case with extreme fluctuations in sugar readings. Ever since then, I have been juggling constantly with various aspects of my lifestyle whether it is exercise, my diet and insulin intake. Forget managing even minimizing the range of my sugar fluctuations has been a very difficult task.

Then one fine day, God must have realised enough is enough, lets give this guy a little break and finally I met Sheryl. A dietitian, nutritionist and I must say a genius in her own right for the work she does – a ready reckoner on diabetes.

Working with Sheryl is systematic. A person very easily available on phone anytime of the day and I mean it. I don't want to delve into details but various aspects like carb counts, diet chart, insulin intake, with realistic & achievable targets, helping my wife with different cuisines of low glycemic index and above all putting our anxiety at ease. This was all made very easy.

IN THE END I CAN VERY WELL SAY THAT SHE IS MY GOD MOTHER.

– Manish Lakhi,
Director, Lakhi Group, Mumbai

I have juvenile diabetes from the age of ten. I also have hypothyrodism, PCOD, and hypertension. I had a still born baby in my first pregnancy and was referred to Sheryl by my doctor when I learned I was pregnant. My HbA1c was 8.4% which means my sugars were not well controlled and could cause complications in pregnancy if I didn't control it well. Sheryl was always there guiding me on what to eat, how to do carbohydrate counting, choosing the right foods when eating out. With her help and guidance I managed my pregnancy well and gave birth to a bonny boy without any problems. My HbA1c when I delivered was 7% and my doctor was very happy. I also lost weight post pregnancy and often have my friends asking me how I managed to do it with my busy social lifestyle. Sheryl has been my living angel in my journey of life, dealing with diabetes and during my most adorable phase – my pregnancy. I have recommended Sheryl to many of my friends who are battling against weight and diabetes.

– **Riddhi Furia,**
Entrepreneur, Mumbai

At the start of 2019, I was concerned about my mommy weight post pregnancy and in addition had a few health scares. I consulted Sheryl and it was all about diet, exercise and finding my balance. The constant monitoring, prodding, pushing, scolding has resulted in me moving from 92.6kg to 75.8 kg in 9 months. The good news is that it's sustainable and the effects are lasting. No yo yo diets no supplements no extreme exercise. Thanks so so much team NHS.

– **Gita Rajagopal,**
Consultant, New Delhi

The best thing we liked about the consult was the one-on-one daily approach to living a better life with Type1 diabetes.

Sheryl has a fantastic patient outlook and led us on a healthy path which should have been clearer years ago.

Fortunately, now that we've been trained, we know better how to deal with T1D with respective to its relation to food.

The consultations lead us to a better lifestyle. Timely eating habits, better diets, insulin management & daily clarifications of doubts made us wiser.

Kudos to NHS for this special consultation on T1D management with respective to food.

Although we've been a Type 1 diabetes family for a decade now, I believe the lives of all three of our daughters are on a healthy path. Please keep on doing the good work.

Appreciate all that you've done. Cheers!

– Pavanbir Singh,
Proud Father to three type 1 daughters, Mumbai

Clarity, time and effort from the health coaches cleared so many doubts and we understood the importance and sensitivity attached with tackling being parents of a type 1 logically, positively and with a 'can do' rather than 'not do' attitude.

The consultation helped us get the sugar levels corrected. Team NHS has always been swift in guiding and handholding me to understand better that rather than just treat insulin as a medicine which you take 3 times a day made me understand the importance of understanding insulin requirements and then administering it.

Team NHS is doing a fantastic job. When it comes to our children, we as parents obviously become extremely sensitive – the most important contribution of NHS being the guidance from the team. For this team it was not a one-off consultation, they were completely involved to help us move in the right direction. This association has impacted us as a family positively – Sheryl every time I give her insulin and I'm thinking how many units my daughter says mama what did Sheryl ma'am say when in doubt give less. Superb team, keep up the good work.

– Pooja Pagdiwala,
Mother of Aarna Pagdiwala, Mumbai

When I was asked to visit NHS, I wondered how it would all go about. But on my visit the consultation time given and the depth in which all details about not only my eating habits but my other medications and exercise were noted meticulously left me impressed. The meal plan was simply superb. All macro and micro nutrients were taken care of and changes in eating pattern were also suggested. I was made to feel at ease. The insulin dose was readjusted. Slowly I have started to feel like my old self again. The heaviness which I used to feel on my face and abdomen has reduced and in 2 months my sugars which used to fluctuate are settling down reducing my insulin dose by nearly 50%. My wife and sister too are trying to follow the pattern of eating; my wife has lost 2 kgs. I would like to thank team NHS in general and Sheryl in particular for the scientific guidance and moral support extended to follow the same. I will always recommend NHS to anyone who wishes to lead a healthy lifestyle.

– Uday Baxi,
Businessman, Gujarat

Made in the USA
Middletown, DE
09 October 2020